CARING FOR
IN HOS

Parents and Nurs

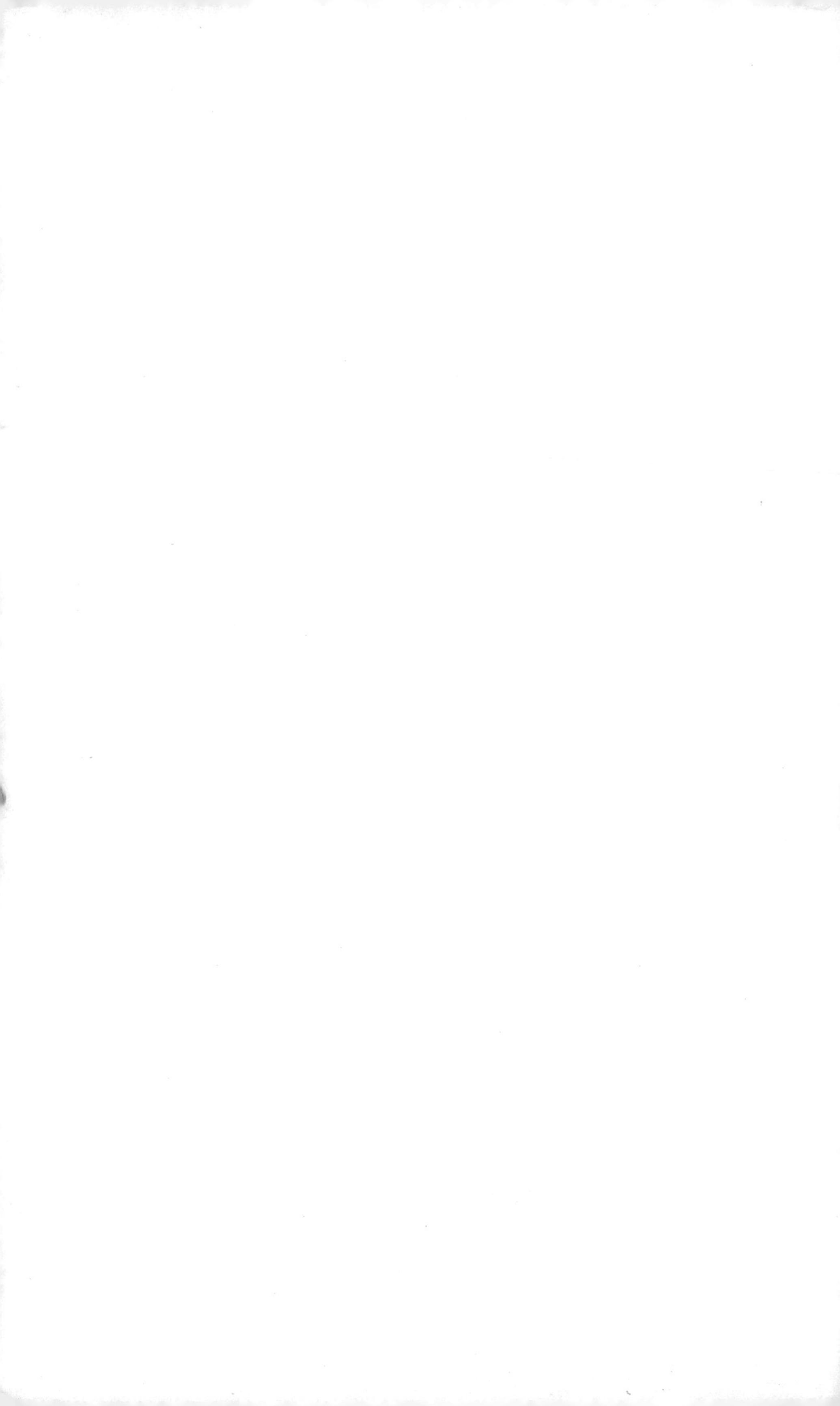

CARING FOR CHILDREN IN HOSPITAL

Parents and Nurses in Partnership

JEAN CLEARY BA
Formerly Senior Research Officer, Institute of Health Care Studies, University College of Swansea;
Department of Child Health, University of Wales College of Medicine

With chapters contributed by Chris Bromley, Imelda Charles-Edwards and Suzanne Goodband with Karen Jennings

Foreword by

SUE BURR MA RSCN RGN RHV RNT
Adviser in Paediatric Nursing, Royal College of Nursing, London

SCUTARI PRESS
London

Scutari Press is a division of Scutari Projects Ltd, the publishing company of the Royal College of Nursing, London.

First published 1992

British Library Cataloguing in Publication Data

Cleary, Jean
Caring for children in hospital – parents and nurses in partnership.
I. Title
362.1083

ISBN 1–871364–67–1

Typeset by Alden Multimedia of Northampton

Printed and bound by Unwin Brothers Ltd.,
The Gresham Press, Old Woking, Surrey GU22 9LH
A Member of the Martins Printing Group

Contents

Contributors		vii
Foreword		ix
Preface		xi
Acknowledgements		xiii
Chapter 1	Introduction – Parents and Children in Hospital	1
Chapter 2	Life on Central Ward: Nurses, Patients and Parents	19
Chapter 3	Setting up the Care-by-Parent Scheme	37
Chapter 4	Care-by-Parent Begins: Life in Three Care Groups	48
Chapter 5	Parents' Experience of Participation and Care-by-Parent	68
Chapter 6	Nurses' Attitudes to the Care-by-Parent Scheme	83
Chapter 7	Developments in the Cardiff Care-by-Parent Scheme *Chris Bromley*	95
Chapter 8	The Philosophy of Care-by-Parent and the Curriculum *Imelda Charles-Edwards*	108
Chapter 9	Parent Care: a US Experience in Indianapolis *Suzanne Goodband with Karen Jennings*	114
Chapter 10	Care-by-Parent – the Basis and the Options	127
Appendix		146
Index		175

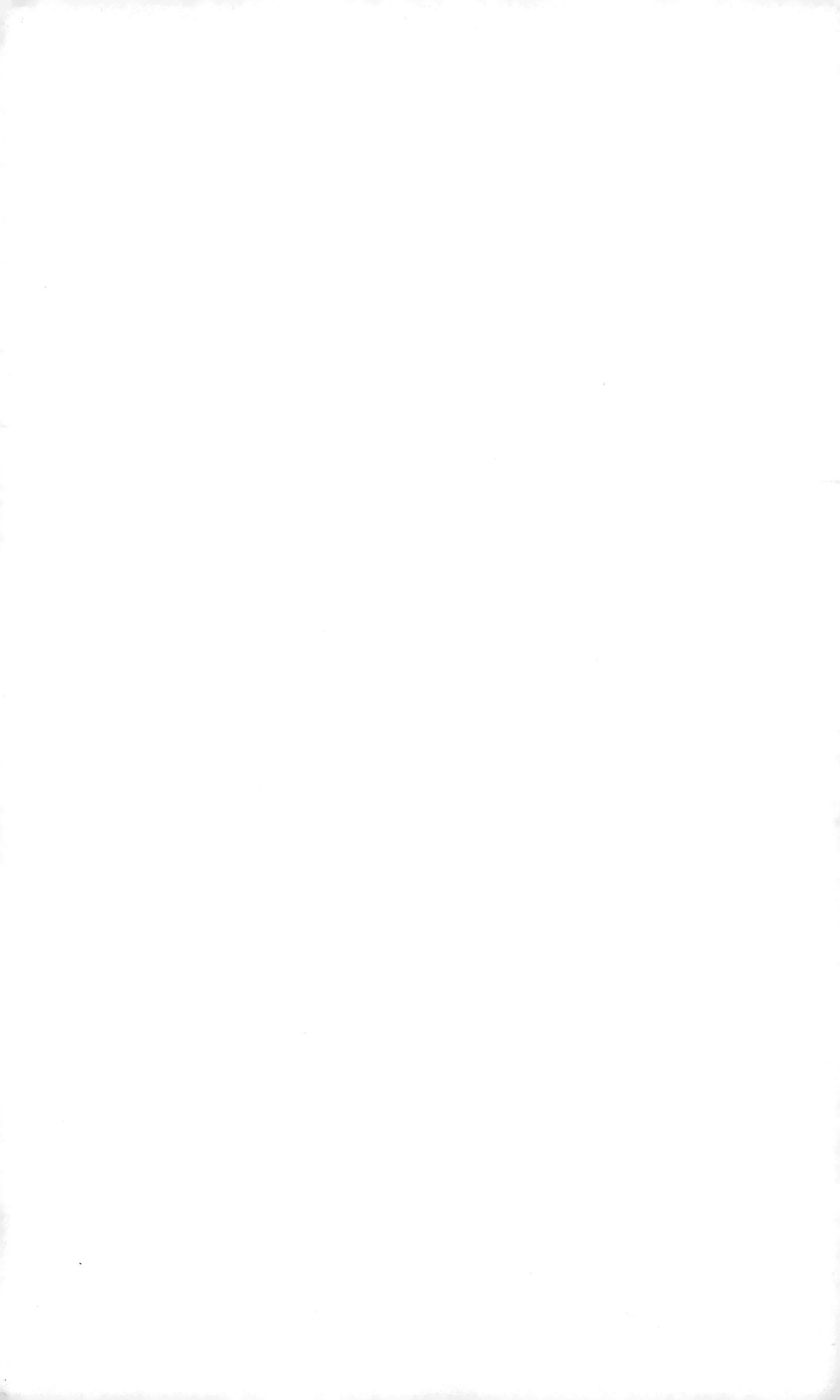

Contributors

CHRIS BROMLEY RSCN RGN

Ward Sister, Child Health Unit, Leicester Royal Infirmary

IMELDA CHARLES-EDWARDS MA, RSCN, RGN, RNT, DipEd, DipN

Assistant Director of Nurse Education, Charles West School of Nursing, The Hospital for Sick Children, Great Ormond Street, London

SUZANNE GOODBAND RSCN, RGN, DipN

Head of Provider Development, East Anglian Regional Health Authority

KAREN JENNINGS RN, MSN

Formerly Director of the Parent Care Unit, James Whitcomb Riley Hospital for Children, Indianapolis

Foreword

Life on the ward for children and their families is, surprisingly, an aspect of care that staff of all disciplines often know very little about, yet surely an understanding of what really occurs is crucial to the provision of both appropriate care and facilities for children and their families in hospital.

The research which forms the basis for this book is a welcome addition to previous studies from the Medical Sociology Research Centre and the Institute of Health Care Studies, University College of Swansea. In the decade that has passed since previous studies were published, hospital care, like many aspects of health care provision, and indeed, society itself, has changed considerably. The care that children in hospital and their families receive must reflect these wider influences, in addition to those resulting from clinical advances and developments within nursing.

Changes in practice include extending the nursing role to one in which nurses work more closely with parents who are active and informed partners in care. This is not a new role for nurses, but a change in emphasis from the primary role of doing to that of educating and supporting patients and their families, particularly parents, who undertake varying degrees of patient care. To be successful, any partnership must be adaptable, flexible and supportive, and good communication between the parties is crucial. Poor communication can be disastrous, not only in clinical terms, but also by parents feeling that they are not trusted, as every move is monitored, that they are in competition with other parents who have been trusted with specific tasks, or, as sometimes already happens with resident parents, that they are abandoned by the nursing staff.

Children and their parents are individuals with individual and constantly changing needs. Parents who may be confidently and competently providing a substantial portion of their child's care may feel unable to continue when circumstances change. This may be due to a deterioration in their child's condition or to a totally unrelated event involving work or other family members. Nurses must be able to identify clues and change the balance of the partnership, assuming more or less of the provision of care as is appropriate at the time.

Successful parent–nurse partnerships do not just happen. As for most things in life, adequate and appropriate preparation, as well as commitment and continuity, are necessary. In addition, nurses require considerable skills and experience in both nursing children and educating and supporting family members. Primary nursing provides a way for both the primary nurse and associate nurses to enhance their skills, and it should also reduce communication difficulties between members of the partnership: it should be considered by those who wish to develop further the parent–nurse partnership in care as established in Cardiff.

Caring for Children in Hospital identifies many common reasons why innovative nursing developments which will enhance the quality of patient care often encounter difficulties. The inclusion of a chapter on curriculum planning acknowledges that knowledge is the forerunner of changing attitudes, and hence behaviour.

In some paediatric wards, real partnership between parents and nurses has been integrated into practice for many years. Unfortunately, wards remain in which parents are only tolerated and nurses demonstrate little insight into the needs of children or their families. This wide disparity is a cause for concern.

This book provides a much-needed insight into life on the ward for children in hospital and their families, and should stimulate the renewal of activities which will enable every child and family to benefit from parents and nurses working in partnership. Family-centred care with parents as active partners with nurses must be the basis of the philosophy of care for all paediatric wards.

SUE BURR
1992

Preface

The care of children in hospital has changed profoundly during the last 25 years. The nursing profession has recognised the importance of children's psychosocial needs, as well as their physical care; the greatest of these needs is to maintain close contact with their families, whose presence is now expected and welcomed. Parents are encouraged to collaborate and participate in the nursing care of their child. This kind of involvement reaches its maximum in care-by-parent schemes and units. The idea has developed in North America, but with roots in both Europe and the Third World. When the University Hospital of Wales decided to introduce its own scheme, Peter Gray, Professor of Child Health, was convinced that it was essential that this new development in care should be carefully monitored, both for its own sake and for the benefit of other hospitals which might wish to adopt the plan. This book is, first and foremost, a record of the setting up and early days of the Cardiff Care-by-Parent Scheme, an innovation within the National Health Service, without the use of additional resources.

However, most children in hospital will continue to be nursed in the more conventional way and the book also gives an account of the lives such children lead during their stay in the wards. It relates their experiences and the part played in them by staff, family and other patients.

Both of these aspects of the study will have significance for those who plan, administer and take part in the care of children within institutions of many kinds as well as those who are considering a career in these areas. This includes doctors, general and paediatric nurses, nursery nurses, managers, teachers, playworkers, the ancillary professions and those involved in residential care. Groups concerned with the welfare of children in hospital or with particular clinical conditions, and those who wish to promote the partnership of parents with professional carers and educators, will find *Caring for Children in Hospital* of great use.

The book's background is as a research project lying broadly within the field of medical sociology, which will be of interest to those whose area of study includes nursing, innovation and institutions, the professions and children. It follows in the Swansea tradition of research on children in hospital, inspired by Margaret Stacey, now Emeritus Professor of Sociology at the University of Warwick. It is essentially an observer's book which demonstrates methods of studying a complex situation by non-participants. It uses both structured and subjective accounts, which rely on recording what was seen, rather than getting participants' accounts which reflect their purposes and perspectives. These methods yield a wealth of both quantitative and qualitative data for analysis. The data are complemented by material which includes the views and experience of those involved, collected through interviews, questionnaires and informal discussions with mothers, fathers, nurses, doctors, other staff and some of the older children.

This is the first comprehensive study of children in hospital in Britain since the earlier work from Swansea, published in *Hospitals, Children and their Families* (1977), *Social Relations and Innovation* (1977) and *Beyond Separation* (1979) (all published by Routledge & Kegan Paul) and Pamela Hawthorn's *'Nurse, I Want My Mummy!'* (RCN, 1974). There are accounts by participants of the work of some of the North American units, and some surveys, but nothing based on systematic and prolonged observation, which is the unique contribution of the Cardiff study.

JEAN CLEARY
1992

Acknowledgements

My thanks are due to many people for support and cooperation during the progress of this work. First and foremost, my thanks to go Peter Gray, Emeritus Professor of Child Health in the University of Wales College of Medicine, and Mai Davies, Nursing Officer (Paediatrics) in the University Hospital of Wales, who believed in the Care-by-Parent Scheme and who were prepared to take the risks associated with innovation and allow the disruption that a research team can cause. Their support was constant and unstinting.

I must express my gratitude to the Leverhulme Trust for the major funding which made the project possible, and to the Jane Hodge Foundation, which also gave financial support. Thanks go, too, to Professor Bill Williams, Director of the Institute of Health Care Studies in the University College of Swansea, who provided me with an academic base, even when the money ran out. The project could not have gone forward without the cooperation of Mrs Annette Watkin, who was Director of Nursing Services at UHW at the time.

I owe an immense personal debt to Margaret Stacey, Emeritus Professor of Sociology at the University of Warwick, who gave me the chance to return to a research career and introduced me to this fascinating and important area – the lives of children in hospital (and the fate of good intentions in institutions).

Thanks are due to all those who served as members of the Steering Committee at various times. I should like to mention particularly the work of the late Marion Ferguson. David Hall, with whom I had worked in the earlier Swansea studies but who now lectures at the University of Liverpool, was also a member of the Committee and always gave his time and good counsel whenever it was needed.

Billie Shepperdson, Bill Bytheway and Roy Mapes, Emeritus Professor of Medical Sociology, are other colleagues who must be mentioned with gratitude, always willing to be treated as sounding boards when ideas needed trying out, or to give advice when asked.

The work of data collection relied heavily upon the skill and good sense of the observers, who were prepared to put up with 6 a.m. starts and midnight finishes to their working day, as well as coping with schedules and coding, while trying to be almost invisible. My heartfelt thanks go to Christine

Bennett, Joan Edwards, Christine Pavelin and Greta Thomas, who worked at both stages of the observations; Maureen Hedley Clarke and Linda Snell at the first stage; and Sheila Jennings and Shelagh Williams at the second. In addition, Greta Thomas carried out many of the post-discharge interviews.

I must also thank Ming Shu Lee and Jacqueline Saunders, of the University of Wales Institute of Science and Technology, whose dissertations I have drawn on in chapters 5 and 6, and John Wiley & Sons Ltd for permission to include my Parents Post-discharge Questionnaire, first published in Seedhouse & Cribb (1989), *Changing Ideas in Health Care*. Thanks also to the RCN Society of Paediatric Nursing for permission to quote from *Standards of Care: Paediatric Nursing* (1990).

There must be special mention of the work of Sister Carol Eden, who got Care-by-Parent going on the wards almost singlehanded, and Dr Clive Sainsbury, who gave it valuable support and foresaw some of its problems. The most important people on the wards, of course, were the children and their parents, who put up with being watched almost day and night (particularly those who were taking on the responsibility for nursing tasks for the first time) in a strange place while they were worried about their sick children. Thanks also to all the staff on the wards, who cooperated with the research team and adopted the new style of work.

I should like to thank my collaborators, who have taken the time to contribute their own expertise to the volume: Chris Bromley, Imelda Charles-Edwards, Suzanne Goodband and Karen Jennings. Finally, I must express my sincere gratitude to Carol Cook, who typed the original draft and several revisions, and also to Carol Johnston, who has helped me come to terms with the word processor.

JC

1

Introduction – Parents and Children in Hospital

The attitudes of health-care workers have changed in the last 25 years, as they have become more sensitive to the emotional and social needs of child patients and their families. More importantly, their practices have changed so that they are more responsive to these needs, particularly recognising the importance of maintaining close contact between children and their families.

I first became aware of the effects of hospitalisation on children when working in a general practitioner's surgery in the 1950s. Visiting in the local hospital was extremely restricted, especially for children under 5 years old, and mothers would try to comfort themselves with the idea that the child 'was in the best place'. The doctor might appear to agree, but privately complained that his efforts to build a relationship of trust with child patients could be ruined by a stay in hospital – 'they scream at the sight of a white coat'.

The desirability of visiting children in hospital was first officially acknowledged in 1950, but the most important recognition of their social and psychological needs occurred in 1956 when the Platt Committee was set up. The publication of its report, *The Welfare of Children in Hospital* (1959), marked a watershed in thinking on the subject. It covered most non-clinical aspects of the lives of children in hospital.

HISTORICAL BACKGROUND OF CARE

In the early 19th century children were rarely admitted to hospital. When they were, they usually had only their mothers to look after them, since the nursing of the period was unskilled, medicine in general lacked a sound theoretical base and paediatrics as a discipline did not exist. The first effective health measures affecting children's care came in the field of public health, particularly from the provision of a clean water supply.

The next influential factors were the developments of anaesthesia and antisepsis, which in turn demanded trained, skilled nurses. With the work of

Pasteur and others on the causes and spread of disease, hospitals became places where people got better rather than died. The climate of opinion about hospital care, including that for children, consequently changed, and White Franklin (1964) says that 38 children's hospitals opened in Britain between 1852 and 1888. Although some authorities, like the surgeon Cooper Forster (1860), stressed children's need for the 'careful and kindly attention of a loving nurse' and 'every kind of amusement', the absence of powerful anti-infective drugs meant that the emphasis of care lay on physical aspects – fresh air, cleanliness and suitable diet – during admissions which could last months if not years, in hospitals built in healthy but remote places. Children were strictly supervised by nurses whose own working and social lives were governed by a thousand rules and regulations and who were also influenced by contemporary ideas on child rearing.

Normal child care, like nursing, became the province of professionals and experts. 'Mothercraft' and 'scientific' child rearing instructed mothers to feed and handle their babies briefly, sticking rigidly to a timetable, and leaving them alone – preferably out of doors – for the rest of the time. Crying was to be ignored and displays of affection avoided – 'Never hug and kiss them, never let them sit in your lap' (Watson 1928). If the child was not healthy, happy and well adjusted, it was, of course, the mother's fault.

Separation from the family and multiple handling, resulting in lack of attachment, which today would be regarded as totally unacceptable, were considered good in themselves. Obviously, visiting children in hospital could not be encouraged, because they became upset and wept when their visitors left. It was said as late as 1940 (in the *Lancet*) that 'the child does not need visitors in the same way as does the adult patient', and only selfish and over-anxious parents would object to the severe visiting restrictions. In any case, the cost and difficulties of travelling to distant hospitals meant that the poor, whose children were still the vast majority of patients, could only visit infrequently. The child whose behaviour was disturbed when he came home from hospital was packed off again to convalescence, often even further from home (Edelston 1943).

On the positive side, immunisation programmes were making headway against infectious disease, and some pioneers found that there was a place for mothers (at least) in the lives of children in hospital.

The period of the Second World War affected the situation in two important ways. First, it provided massive evidence on the effects of separation: in England, on families split by war service and evacuation; in Europe, from children made homeless by battles and bombing or found in concentration and displaced persons' camps (Bowlby 1952, Robertson 1958, Wicks 1988). Second, it saw the development of powerful new drugs, the sulphanilamides and the antibiotics. With these, many diseases became much less dangerous and cures took a fraction of the time – days rather than months.

Against this background of new pharmaceutical weaponry, which allowed the consideration of the child's social and psychological needs (since survival was rarely in doubt), and a developing understanding of those needs, the new National Health Service in Britain set up the Committee on the Welfare of Children in Hospital, with Sir Harry Platt as chairman. Its report was published in 1959.

PLATT'S RECOMMENDATIONS

Platt's first recommendation in the Report was a general one about paying attention to the emotional and mental needs of children in hospital; the second was that children should not be admitted to hospital at all if it could possibly be avoided. These recommendations were followed by details about the conditions in which children should be nursed, beginning with 'children and adolescents should not be nursed in adult wards'. The most controversial proposals were unrestricted visiting for parents, by which they meant 'at any reasonable hour' and at the discretion of the ward sister, and the admission of mothers (no mention of fathers) with their children, especially those under 5 years of age. Both resident and visiting parents should 'help as much as possible with the care of the child'. The Ministry of Health (as it was then called) adopted the Platt Report, and its recommendations became policy.

IMPLEMENTING PLATT

Keeping children out of hospital

Given that 'Children . . . should only be admitted to hospital when the medical treatment they require cannot be given in other ways, without real disadvantage', the Report encouraged day-care and home nursing schemes. Change has proceeded slowly towards this and, more than 15 years on, another major report said that paediatrics should be less hospital-bound and commented on the slow development of day-care and domiciliary paediatric nursing services. This was the Court Report, from the Child Health Services Committee (1976). It stressed 'the obvious advantages of avoiding separation from the family and home or shortening the length of stay in hospital.'

In some areas of the country, for example Southampton, and for some clinical conditions, like diabetes, there has been considerable expansion of day-care and domiciliary services. With the passage of another 15 years, much more consideration is being given to domiciliary paediatric nursing services, both as the rational consequence of involving parents in the care of their children in hospital and from the current emphasis on care in the community (including economic constraints).

Children's admissions and readmissions

Are the numbers of children being admitted to hospital going down in response to the recognition of the importance of keeping them out of hospital and to the expansion of domiciliary services and day-case treatment? This question is more complicated than it first appears. The best figures available only go up to 1985 and derive from returns made by health authorities to the Department of Health and Social Security (DHSS).

Since that date a new system has been introduced, which replaces the collation of data from the returns. The Körner system, named after the chairperson of the Steering Group on Health Services Information, produces statistics from patient-level data. A minimum data-set has been laid down, which can be extended to meet local needs. The aim is to produce data which are accurate, relevant and timely; derived as a by-product of operational data handling where possible; and used to inform management decisions. Unfortunately, lack of financial resources and, technical expertise has delayed the production of some statistics and, so far, children's non-psychiatric admissions have not been distinguished from the total (Department of Health 1991).

Figure 1.1 shows that the general tendency of child hospital admissions in England is upward and stresses the fact that the youngest age group (0–4 years) is by far the most likely to be admitted. Statistics for Wales (Figure 1.2, p.6) are not so detailed but show a similar upward trend. Day cases are not included in these figures, but Figure 1.3, (p.7) shows that, in England, their numbers are also rising, and much more dramatically. The rates used take account of variations in the size of the population in the age groups but one important factor is missing: the statistics refer to discharges from, or 'spells' in, hospital and not to individual children, who may have been admitted more than once. This means that it cannot be assumed that the rates show just how the numbers of child patients are rising.

Children who have chronic conditions are likely to be admitted more often than others and, frequently, more than once in a year: asthma, cystic fibrosis and cancer are obvious examples. Unfortunately, data on readmission rates are not collected nationally, but only on occasion by interested hospitals or districts or as part of other research.

Cohort studies which have followed up all the children born in a single week over many years have looked at various aspects of health and development. A study of children born in 1970 shows that the proportion hospitalised by the age of 5 was 25.5%, compared with 18.5% of a 1946 cohort: more than a quarter of the 1970 children who had been in hospital had been in more than once, and one child with spina bifida had had 33 admissions (Golding & Haslum 1986).

The General Household Survey, another source of a wide range of information about the life of a sample of households, began asking in 1983 about hospital admissions. In 1985 about one tenth of the under-5s surveyed had been in-patients during the preceding year, but these (approximately) 170 children had had about 240 admissions. Among the older children, up to and

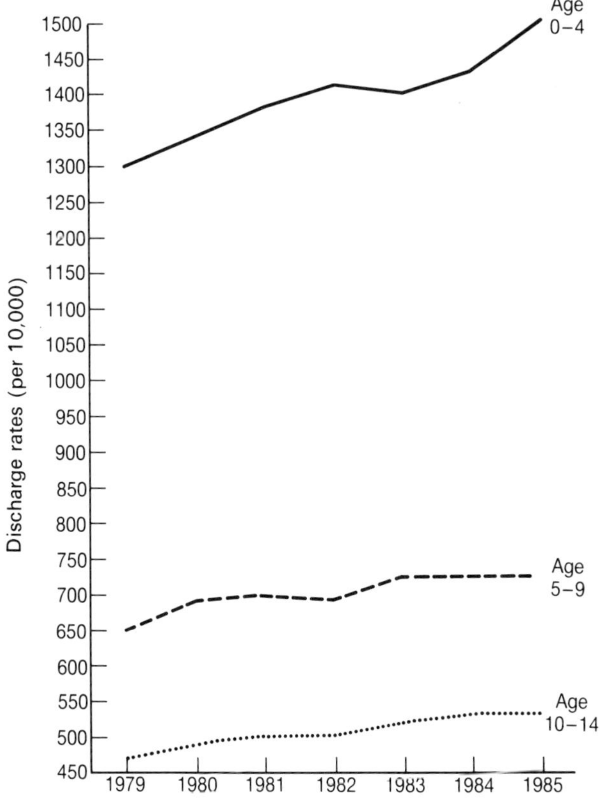

Based on data from Health and Personal Social Services Statistics (DHSS)

Figure 1.1 Discharges from hospital: rates per 10,000 population by age group – England

including 15 years of age, the proportion that had gone into hospital was lower – about one in 16 – with approximately 240 children sharing 300 admissions. In the same year, in one London district, nearly 15% of child patients had been admitted more than once.

'More than once' obviously does not indicate precisely how often any one child might have been admitted. In a study carried out in the children's wards of a general hospital in the early 1970s, the analysis showed that one fifth of the children who were readmitted within the year were in hospital more than twice – usually three, four or five times (the total number of children in the wards was over 1000). In the Cardiff study there have been individual children with metabolic disorders or problematic hydrocephalus whose admissions were well into double figures by the time they were 2 or 3 years old – they might be called veterans. One mother reckoned that her daughter

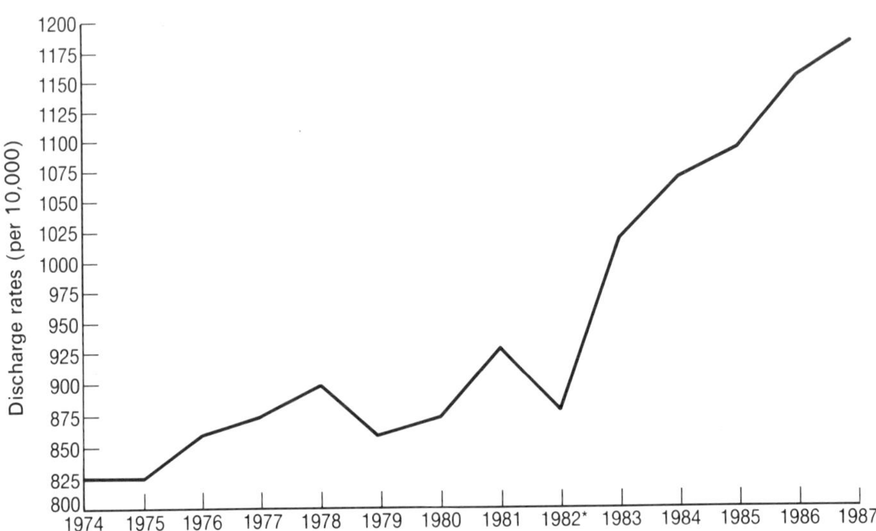

Based on data from Health and Personal Social Service Statistics for Wales (Welsh Office)
*Figures for 1982 were affected by industrial action

Figure 1.2 Discharges from hospital: rates per 10,000 population – Wales, age 0–14 years

had been in hospital with her rare blood condition 46 times by the time she was 5.

However, the figures do not simply reflect the obvious point that some children inevitably go into hospital more often than others. They demonstrate changes in practice as well. Nowadays, paediatricians and other specialists, such as orthopaedic surgeons, are reluctant to keep children in hospital throughout a long course of treatment or investigation, as they might once have done; instead, they send them home in non-active phases of treatment, for breaks or for trial runs. Each hospital episode may be (but is not always) treated as a new admission.

Discharges from paediatrics wards in the Oxford region have been examined in detail by Hill (1989). Having considered all the alternative explanations – the increase in readmission rate in general and, in particular, in that of babies who previously might not have survived, she concludes that lower threshold levels for admission are being used. Despite Platt and Court, children are more, rather than less, likely to become in-patients, although the stays are for shorter periods. There are also children categorised as 'ward attenders' who are not formally admitted. They are described as 'hidden children' (Thornes 1988), spending fairly brief periods, probably less than 2 hours, on the wards. The main reasons for their presence are the need for a second opinion, the performance of a test or because the parents are

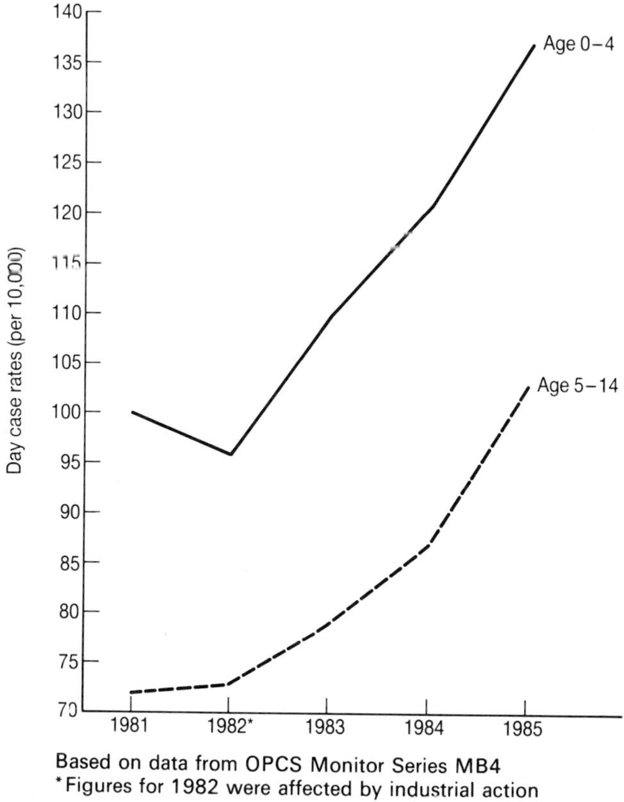

Figure 1.3 Day cases: rates per 10,000 population – England

worried about some deterioration in condition, the fit of a caliper or a broken plaster. They often form between 11 and 20% of the ward's patients, having a considerable effect upon the workload of nurses, who provide education and support, and putting pressure on space and facilities.

Children in adult wards

Both Platt and Court, as well as the circular *Hospital Facilities for Children* (DHSS & Welsh Office 1971), recommend that children should not be nursed in adult wards and that they should be in the general care of a paediatrician. Analysis of the 1984 figures – 35 years after Platt – shows that many children are still admitted to adult wards (Table 1.1, p.8) and to specialties other than paediatrics (Table 1.2, p.8).

Hill's (1989) study also shows that although admissions to paediatric wards had risen over 10 years, they were still only 38% of the total for children under 15.

Table 1.1 Death and discharge from adult or mixed wards

Age (years)	% of child in-patients
0–4	10.1[1]
5–11	21.8[1]
12–16	61.8[2]

[1] Based on 8 English regions n = 109,719
[2] Based on 7 English regions n = 106,836

Hospital admission and its effects

Bearing all these factors in mind, it is clear that some of the increase in admissions relates to children whose health means that they will frequently be patients, including those with conditions that used to prove fatal. However, the steady rise in the figures also suggests that children are not so far being kept out of hospital in significant numbers. The most common reasons for admission for children are accidents and the need for surgery – the avoidance of admission for these cases is difficult. The youngest age group are admitted more often than others and it is this age group which has been shown to be the most vulnerable to the trauma of hospitalisation in the past (Douglas 1975).

A more recent cohort study from New Zealand (Shannon et al 1984) suggests that modern paediatric practices, unrestricted visiting and liberal facilities for mothers to stay mean that few in the age group 0–4 years showed post-hospital behaviour problems at the age of 6, although there was some

Table 1.2 Death and discharge by specialty[1]

Specialty	% of child in-patients
Paediatrics	35.6
Special care babies	7.7
Paediatric surgery	1.5
Total	44.8
General surgery	14.8
ENT surgery	13.9
Traumatic and orthopaedic surgery	10.5
Remaining specialties	15.9
Total	55.1

[1] n = 815,165; excludes Wessex and Special Health Authorities

association noted between level of disturbance and length of stay. This, to some extent, confirms that the key to successful, non-damaging hospitalisation lies in involving parents.

Psychosocial factors and research

How were Platt's recommendations about parents implemented? The evidence from the 1960s and 70s suggests that in most cases it was with reluctance. Robertson's book *Hospitals and Children: a Parent's-eye View* (1962) collates the experiences of many families, who found that 'at any reasonable hour' and 'at the discretion of the ward sister' could be interpreted in ways which defeated the intentions of the policy makers. Parliamentary questions to the Minister of Health received encouraging replies about unrestricted visiting, but these were not borne out by the results of surveys carried out by the National Association for the Welfare of Children in Hospital (NAWCH), a pressure group set up in 1961. The official figure given in 1966 for the level of unrestricted visiting (85%) was not achieved until 1982. Accommodation for mothers was granted grudgingly, if at all, and practically never offered unless requested. Many nurses remained unconvinced by ideas associated with psychoanalysis, and were hostile to breaking with past practice, particularly as there was seldom any attempt to explain changes to the staff on the ward.

During the same period, research was being carried out on both sides of the Atlantic on ways to improve the situation for child patients, for instance having mothers to stay with them (Brain & Maclay 1968) or providing mothers with accurate information and support (Skipper & Leonard 1968). Both these options proved to have physical as well as psychological benefits for the children, when compared with control groups.

A study of a group in late adolescence who had been followed up since their birth in 1946 (Douglas 1975) suggested that those who had been in hospital for one long or several short stays before the age of 5 were more likely to show behavioural disturbance and poor reading ability. These children would have been admitted at a time when visiting was very restricted. A second cohort study of 10-year-olds (Quinton & Rutter 1976), whose hospital experience would have been after the publication of the Platt Report, showed a similar pattern of disturbance, but the authors considered that this could be due to social factors in their background.

The Swansea studies

During the 1960s, the first series of studies on children in hospital, directed by Margaret Stacey (Stacey et al 1970), was set up in Swansea. Children who were to be admitted for tonsillectomy were assessed beforehand, observed while they were in hospital and followed up for 6 months afterwards. The most striking findings were the proportion of time that children spent alone and unoccupied, the way in which visiting was discouraged – although visitors were still the children's most important contacts – and that all the children were disturbed to some extent by the admission. A linked project reported on the attitudes to hospital and experiences related to visiting of a large group of parents. An unrelated study (Hawthorn 1974), set up by the Royal College of Nursing (RCN), largely confirmed the Swansea observations.

In the second series of Swansea studies a multidisciplinary team examined:

1. the concept of vulnerability;
2. the lives of long-stay patients, mainly orthopaedic;
3. the effects of putting playleaders on ordinary acute children's wards.

The team, of which I was a member, included sociologists, anthropologists and psychologists, and again relied principally on observational research methods. The results of our work was published in *Beyond Separation* (Hall & Stacey 1979).

Brown's vulnerability study (1979) showed a correlation between behaviour on the ward and post-hospital disturbance, linked to the style of family life – one psychological test used seemed to have considerable value as a predictor.

The study of young long-stay patients (Pill & Jacobs 1979) discovered that this was, at the time, a very small category. Instead there were the children who had frequent short admissions, which disrupted their normal lives and education, without ensuring continuity in their hospital lives. They suffered particularly from the immobility their treatment involved and the ensuing boredom.

Clough (1979) studied a group of long-stay patients: teenage girls having surgery for scoliosis. Psychological measures were employed to examine their reactions to their treatment and what it meant to them.

The aim of Hall (1979) and Cleary's playleader study was to find out whether having a playleader on the ward improved the lives of ordinary child patients: the findings were reported in *Social Relations and Innovation: Changing the State of Play in Hospitals* (Hall 1977). Children did lead more normal active lives and parents were enthusiastic about their work, but nursing staff and hospital teachers were not sure how to relate to their new colleagues. The observations also highlighted continuing problems with unrestricted visiting and the effects of task assignment as a style of organising nursing work (Cleary 1977, 1979). Like the Expert Group on Play for Children in Hospital (DHSS 1976), the researchers concluded that professional playleaders were essential, but the decision of the DHSS – which had funded this and all the Swansea research – was that, on economic grounds, responsibility for play should remain with the nurses.

The findings on visiting and nursing style also formed the background to the present study.

EXPERIENCE OF HOSPITAL

A first-hand account

There are few first-hand accounts from young children who underwent the old-style lengthy hospital admissions. One harrowing account of an extreme case was published in the *Lancet* in 1949, and refers to a period before the First World War. It is noteworthy because the author is concerned very little with his physical suffering but rather with his emotional pain, particularly the effects of catastrophic separation on the rest of his life. He begins:

> A severe knee injury at the age of six brought me to an orthopaedic institution some hundreds of miles away from home [a tubercular infection of the joint flared up]. My leg was encased in plaster and I was left at the hospital for just over three years. The desperate homesickness and misery of the early weeks gave way to indifference and boredom . . . Looking back on this experience from a distance of forty-odd years it is surprising how serene my memories of it are compared with memories of the rest of my childhood. I endured many discomforts, and I lived in perpetual dread of the weekly aspirations of pus which were done through an opening in the plaster; but none of this seems to have left a mark, and I remember my mother's first and only visit far more vividly. It occurred many months after my admission and was evidently not voted a success, for it was not repeated. I can still feel the chill of disappointment at seeing her suddenly in the room, for I could think of absolutely nothing to say to her. The total inadequacy of my emotional response to her shocked me and gave a sense of unreality to our meeting which will haunt me through life. Contact with home had been out of the question at that distance, and the kind of letters that could be written to a child of six provided no link . . .

The distance involved, the length of time his recovery took, and the lack of contact with his family seem in themselves an almost incredible combination of adverse circumstances, but in addition the plaster 'cut me off from every outlet for my physical energies', while his life in a cubicle 'gave practically no scope for self-expression'. His one stroke of good fortune in this solitary confinement was finding a mother figure in the shape of the hospital superintendent, but the strength of this attachment separated him still further from his family and already 'home had become a worry and a source of bewilderment to me'. Obviously, his problems were not going to end with hospitalisation.

> I discovered this on being uprooted a second time, and restored to my home again. All my former insecurities assailed me, for I returned an alien; I held a passport indeed, but it had ceased to be valid long since.

His route to a fairly happy ending lay in academic achievement and putting 'several thousand miles' between himself and his family. He married, which 'completed the emotional cure, so far as this could be done'. He ends by saying that 'a solution to my particular problem in the absence of a good intelligence, I am unable to imagine'. To intelligence, the reader would want to add insight, neither of which are granted to all child patients.

This history is probably just that – history – but it describes the most extreme form of hospitalisation, which went on in a modified way until relatively recently. Separation, remote hospitals and long admissions were often the experience of, for example, boys with Perthes' disease.

The child's experience

Any admission to hospital is full of strangeness to the small child, most child patients being younger than 6 years old. When children go to hospital they are generally feeling ill or are injured – elective admissions form a very small part of the total. When children are ill or hurt at home they generally want, and get, a great deal of attention. The old-fashioned hospital required the child to be handed over, and visiting was kept to a minimum. It was the psychoanalytically-oriented doctors and therapists who first pointed out that, to a small child, this must seem like punishment for some unknown crime. To be taken away from all that is familiar and comforting, to have strangers do bewildering, perhaps painful, things to you and to find that your mother and father, even if they are there, have become inexplicably powerless, instead of taking charge of your life, is 'the world turned upside down'.

Some people found, and still find, these notions about punishment unacceptable by being based on too imaginative a view of the child's thinking. However, recent work, for example that of Brewster (1982), starting from an entirely different theoretical base – Piaget's theories of cognitive development – has shown that children, even up to the age of 5 or 6, regard illness as the result of wrongdoing and painful procedures as punishment for it.

The physical environment is unlike anything children are familiar with. There are different beds, different food, no ordinary arrangement of rooms, times when they have to keep still and times when they have to stay in bed, to say nothing of temperature taking, medication, infusions or traction. Above all, there are strangers, who invade their privacy, wash them, dress them, and tell them what to do. And, despite case assignment or primary nursing, there are still large numbers of strangers involved, dictated by the need for breaks, shift changes, leave, the demands of nurse education and the business of the ward. An example of this concerns Owen, a handicapped 2-year-old in Cardiff, who was being barrier nursed during nearly a week of activity sampling where observations were taken at 20-minute intervals (see Appendix). He was recorded with at least five, and sometimes seven or eight, members of the nursing staff each day. His parents cared for him during their daily visits, but during the week he received care from, at minimum, 16 nurses, as well as from involved medical and ancillary staff.

The parents' experience

Alongside the child's anxiety and distress is the concern of the parents – worry about the condition and its outcome, worry about how the child is being looked after. There is relief when the hospital takes control of a dangerous situation but also feelings of helplessness and failure, even guilt, that the child should have become so ill or suffered such hurt as to need to be taken out of the family's care. Lack of information about what may happen or what the parents can safely do aggravates these feelings.

Currently, about two-thirds of wards for children have completely unrestricted visiting, meaning at any hour of the day or night, while most of the rest permit it for more than 10 hours a day. There may, however, be other kinds of restriction, for example, on the day of the operation or for particular specialties. Practically all wards have facilities for at least some parents to stay overnight, which was another of Platt's proposals, and many offer it as part of the admission routine. It is probably more widely practised than the Committee ever envisaged, since they only referred to the admission of mothers with their children and then particularly 'for the first day or two'. Fathers and other relatives may now share care with the mother, or take over from her all that is involved in being resident with the child. Resident parents generally remain for the whole of the average stay. Changes in society, the increase in fathers' involvement in child care and in mothers' employment outside the home, as well as a keener appreciation of the dangers of separating family members, have, in some ways, overtaken Platt.

When parents are present, particularly in the early stages of an admission, they are frequently unsure of what to do. Is it all right to give the child a drink of water, let him run about, leave the cubicle? Should they go away when staff come to do something: are they not wanted or are they physically in the way? Parents may have only their own childhood experiences to go by and not realise how a parent's role has changed. Conversely, they may find themselves in one of the diminishing number of hospitals which do not give parents any active part in care, and be afraid of overstepping the mark.

Parents have other problems, too, when they are resident or visit for long periods every day. Apart from worries about the rest of the family, they may find boredom and ensuing guilt competing with anxiety. If the child is too ill to want more than a comforting familiar presence, or needs a totally unfamiliar one-to-one concentration on play, the hours may pass very slowly, deprived of all normal responsibilities and occupations. Being resident generally lacks privacy as well – one mother described it as like 'living in a goldfish bowl' – and the accommodation will probably be cramped, possibly uncomfortable and noisy.

IS MORE CHANGE NEEDED?

Although rates of children's admission have not begun to fall, measures have been introduced which could have an effect on the situation. Community paediatric nursing schemes, which are becoming more widespread, mean that not only can some admissions be avoided altogether, but also support and back-up can be given for day-case treatment and very early discharge.

Hospitals, for the most part, welcome parents as visitors or residents, while providing skilled professional nursing care. So, apart from some minor discomforts, is everything for 'the best in the best of all possible worlds'? Is there any need for more change? Parents still report that children are upset in hospital and suffer post-discharge disturbance. Parents themselves have problems with their role in the ward. Some children still spend a great deal of their time in hospital, which might be lessened by some means. Can the situation be improved for parents and children without endangering or hampering the clinical aspects of care? Would the changes adversely affect the nurses' work and job satisfaction? These are questions which the Cardiff project set out to consider.

There are other major questions, for instance whether the numbers of children admitted to non-paediatric wards can be reduced and whether their special needs are being recognised there and when passing through other hospital departments. These require investigation but are outside the scope of this work.

PARENTAL INVOLVEMENT

When the mother and father are involved in the child's nursing care as far as possible, which is found most completely in care-by-parent schemes, changes will follow. The problems do not all disappear, but many of the worries and uncertainties and much of the tedium do. The parent knows what is allowed and what needs to be done and has been taught how to do it and how to record it. When routines can be modified, procedures can be carried out in the manner which suits the individual child best, by the person who knows what that is. Anxiety does not disappear; indeed, carrying out these unfamiliar procedures may increase it, but for nearly every parent the satisfaction of being a well-informed and responsible member of the care team and playing a real part in the child's care more than compensates for this. The child is handled nearly all the time by a familiar care giver, who knows him and his ways better than anyone else, rather than by a succession of strangers, however skilled or well-meaning they may be.

The greater understanding and competence which parents develop by participating in an informed way in care has long-term benefits for the whole family in coping with future episodes of illness, especially where the patient has a chronic condition. At the very least, parents become better judges of the condition and learn when to seek professional help. It may prove possible to cut down the number of admissions to hospital or to reduce their length when more skilled care is available at home, and the child's quality of life will improve.

STAFF EXPERIENCE OF CARE-BY-PARENT

Care-by-parent does not appear to affect the work of children's doctors to any great degree. Paediatricians, in particular, are used to the presence of parents on the ward and to including them in discussions about their children. Better-informed parents will have more useful dialogue with professionals.

Earlier changes had been accepted reluctantly because they had been imposed rather than agreed. There was little understanding of the reasoning behind them or of their impact on the work at ward level. The phrase 'philosophy of care' was not in use at the time the Cardiff Care-by-Parent Scheme was being set up, but the paediatric nursing staff were committed to family-centred care. The new scheme was a further step along this road. Instead of giving all the hands-on care themselves, nurses were to be the teachers of new skills to parents, instructing and guiding them until they had gained sufficient confidence and competence to take on some or all of the nursing care, while providing emotional support throughout their stay. They would be called upon to share their professional knowledge, relinquish some of their authority and lose much of the direct contact with some of their patients, although the ultimate responsibility would still be theirs. They were to become the teachers and counsellors of the natural care givers, planning and demonstrating rather than implementing care. In care-by-parent schemes, recognition is given to the importance of these roles and sufficient time is always made available to carry them out satisfactorily.

Against this background the Cardiff Care-by-Parent Scheme was set up: it was considered essential that research should examine the current situation in a paediatric unit and assess the feasibility and impact of this innovation in nursing practice. This book gives an account of, first, paediatric care in a parent-friendly environment and, second, the effects of the Care-by-Parent Scheme. The research was based chiefly on non-participant observation, from approximately 6.15 a.m. to 11.30 p.m. The techniques, developed from those in the earlier Swansea studies, used precoded schedules of two kinds: activity sampling which produced a series of 'snapshots' of all that was going on in an area, every 20 minutes, and case studies of individual children, who were watched continuously for 5 minutes in every hour. These were supplemented by diaries kept by each observer, post-discharge questionnaires administered to the parents of case study children and a survey of nurses' attitudes before the observations began, as well as many informal discussions with parents, older patients and staff in all disciplines. A letter to parents explained the nature and purpose of the research and asked permission to include their children in it. This and details about the research methods are given in the Appendix. There were two periods of observations, one before the CBP Scheme was set up, which focused on the ordinary life of the Paediatric Unit and the second when the Scheme had been established. Each lasted five weeks. Chapter 2 reports on life in a multibedded room during the first period and Chapter 4 compares three groups of children, mainly infants, during the second period when the Scheme was running.

REFERENCES

Bowlby J (1952) *Maternal Care and Mental Health.* Geneva: World Health Organisation.

Brain DJ & Maclay I (1968) Controlled study of mothers and children in hospital. *British Medical Journal*, **i**: 278–80.

Brewster AB (1982) Chronically ill hospitalized children's concepts of their illness. *Pediatrics*, **69**: 355–62.

Brown BJ (1979) Beyond separation: some new evidence on the impact of brief hospitalisation on young children. In Hall DJ & Stacey M, *Beyond Separation*, pp 18-53. London: Routledge & Kegan Paul.

Child Health Services Committee (1976) *Fit for the Future* (the Court Report). London: DHSS, DES and Welsh Office.

Cleary J (1977) The distribution of nursing attention in a children's ward. *Nursing Times* Occasional Papers, July 14: 93–6.

Cleary J (1979) Demands and responses: the effects of the style of work allocation on the distribution of nursing attention. In Hall DJ & Stacey M, *Beyond Separation*, pp 109–27. London: Routledge & Kegan Paul.

Clough F (1979) The validation of meaning in illness treatment situations. In Hall DJ & Stacey M, *Beyond Separation*, pp 54–81. London: Routledge & Kegan Paul.

Department of Health (1991) *Health and Personal Social Services Statistics for England.* London: Government Statistical Service.

DHSS & Welsh Office (1971) *Hospital Facilities for Children*, HM (71) 22.

Douglas JWB (1975) Early hospital admissions and later disturbances of behaviour and learning. *Developmental Medicine and Child Neurology*, **17**: 456–80.

Edelston H (1943) Separation anxiety in young children. *Genetic Psychology Monographs*, **28**.

Expert Group on Play for Children in Hospital (1976) *Report*, London: DHSS.

Forster J Cooper (1860) *The Surgical Diseases of Children.* London: John W Parker & Son.

Golding J & Haslum M (1986) Hospital admissions. In Butler NR and Golding J (eds.), *From Birth to Five*, pp. 242–54. Oxford: Pergamon.

Hall DJ (1977) *Social Relations and Innovation: Changing the State of Play in Hospitals.* London: Routledge & Kegan Paul.

Hall DJ (1979) On calling for order: aspects of the organisation of patient care. In Hall DJ & Stacey M, *Beyond Separation*, pp 155–78. London: Routledge & Kegan Paul.

Hall DJ & Stacey M (1979) *Beyond Separation.* London: Routledge & Kegan Paul.

Hawthorn PJ (1974) *'Nurse – I Want my Mummy!'.* London: RCN.

Hill AM (1989). Trends in paediatric medical admissions. *British Medical Journal*, **298**: 1479–83.

Jacobs R (1979) The meaning of hospital: denial of emotions. In Hall DJ & Stacey M, *Beyond Separation*, pp 82–108. London: Routledge & Kegan Paul.

Lancet (1949) Hospitalisation in childhood. *Lancet*, June 4: 975–6.

Ministry of Health, Central Health Services Council (1959) *The Welfare of Children in Hospital* (the Platt Report). London: Ministry of Health.

Pill R (1979) Status and career: a sociological approach to the study of child patients. In Hall DJ & Stacey M, *Beyond Separation*, pp 82–108. London: Routledge & Kegan Paul.

Quinton D & Rutter M (1976) Early hospital admissions and subsequent and later disturbances of behaviour: an attempted replication of Douglas' findings. *Developmental Medicine and Child Neurology*, **18**: 447–59.

Robertson J (1958) *Young Children in Hospital*. London: Tavistock Publications.

Robertson J (1962) *Hospitals and Children: a Parent's-eye View*. London: Gollancz.

Shannon FT, Fergusson DM & Dimond ME (1984) Early hospital admissions and subsequent behaviour problems in 6 year olds. *Archives of Disease in Childhood*, **59**: 815–19.

Skipper JK & Leonard RC (1968) Children, stress and hospitalization: a field experiment. *Journal of Health and Social Behaviour*, **9**: 275–87.

Stacey M, Dearden R, Pill R & Robinson D (1970) *Hospitals, Children and their Families: the Report of a Pilot Study*. London: Routledge & Kegan Paul.

Thornes R (1987) *Where are the Children?* London: Caring for Children in the Health Services, c/o NAWCH.

Thornes R (1988) *Hidden Children*. London: Caring for Children in the Health Services, c/o NAWCH.

Watson JB (1928) *Psychological Care of the Infant and Child*. London: Allen & Unwin.

White Franklin A (1964) Children's hospitals. In Poynter FNL (ed.), *The Evolution of Hospitals in Britain*, pp 103–21. London: Pitman.

Wicks B (1988) *No Time to Wave Goodbye: True Stories of Britain's 3,500,000 Evacuees*. London: Bloomsbury.

FURTHER READING

Brandon S (1986) *Children in Hospital: Life is Short and the Art is Long*. London: NAWCH.

Cule J & Turner T (eds.) (1986) *Child Care Through the Centuries*. Cardiff: STS Publishing, for the British Society for the History of Medicine.

Gow M & Atwell J (1980) The role of the children's nurse in the community. *Journal of Pediatric Surgery*, **15**(i): 26–30.

Hardyment C (1983) *Dream Babies: Child Care from Locke to Spock*. London: Jonathan Cape.

Jolly J (1981) *The Other Side of Paediatrics: a Guide to the Everyday Care of Sick Children*. London: Macmillan.

Mead D & Sibert J (1991) *The Injured Child: an Action Plan for Nurses*. London: Scutari Press.

Meadow SR (1969) The captive mother. *Archives of Disease in Childhood*, **9**: 275–87.

Petrillo M & Sanger S (1972) *Emotional Care of Hospitalized Children*. Philadelphia: Lippincott.

Piaget J (1932) *Moral Judgement in Children.* London: Kegan Paul.

Richards MPM (ed.) (1974) *The Integration of a Child into a Social World.* London: Cambridge University Press.

Thornes R (1988) *Parents Staying Overnight with their Children in Hospital.* London: Caring for Children in the Health Services, c/o NAWCH.

2

Life on Central Ward: Nurses, Patients and Parents

The main purpose of the Cardiff project was to establish whether care-by-parent was possible and useful within British NHS hospitals. It was recognised that this option would probably only be feasible in the larger paediatric units and that not every child or every parent could be a candidate for it. Its other aim, therefore, was to provide information which would be relevant to the situation of the majority of child patients. The first set of observations was carried out while the way that the Care-by-Parent Scheme would be run was still under discussion. They would show how the lives of children in hospital had been changed by the implementation of the Platt Report's (Ministry of Health 1959) recommendations, children nursed in the ordinary way, but by nurses to whom Platt's ideas were part of the normal basis of their work, rather than the thunderbolt they appeared at first. It seems likely that the majority of children will always be admitted to multibedded rooms and that their parents will play a minor role in their nursing care. This chapter describes the lives of a group of these children during one week in October.

The University Hospital of Wales was built during the 1960s, on a typical site, on the far side of a motorway-type road. It took over some, but not all, of the functions of the old Cardiff Royal Infirmary (not, for example, accident and emergency) but did not replace it. It is the District General Hospital for parts of South and Mid-Glamorgan and the tertiary centre for many specialties in Wales, as well as housing the University of Wales College of Medicine. The Paediatric Unit therefore takes not only those with the usual run of respiratory and gastroenterological problems or with asthma, hernia and appendicitis, but also children with severe and multiple handicaps, like hydrocephalus, congenital heart disease and cerebral palsy. Two important groups of children, diabetic and paediatric oncology patients, are normally admitted to other hospitals in the area. The reasons why the

Care-by-Parent Scheme began there rather than anywhere else are discussed in the next chapter.

The new Paediatric Unit opened in 1972 and comprises 3 wards. The unit always had unrestricted visiting for parents and other important adults – important to the child that is. Children could visit every day and one adult could stay overnight with any child: there was no age-limit.

North Ward (see Figure 4.1) has 14 cubicles and includes facilities for resident parents as well. The majority of children nursed in the Care-by-Parent Scheme and observed as part of the research were on this ward. Central Ward (Figure 2.1) was mainly for older children with medical conditions, and has 7 cubicles (8 beds) and one 8-bed room. South Ward was primarily surgical and did not join in the Care-by-Parent Scheme during the research phase; it had 2 multibedded rooms and 4 cubicles. There is also a Special Care Baby Unit and a new Paediatric Cardiology Unit: the functions of the other wards have changed somewhat.

The children to be described here were patients in the 8-bed room on Central Ward (C8), where the ordinary routine resembled that of many other hospitals, where staff try to meet the children's psychosocial needs. When parents wanted to stay with their children and there was no cubicle available, this generally meant sleeping in a chair at the bedside or in off-ward accommodation. Parents who were present in the ward were always expected to carry out ordinary basic care: washing, feeding and toileting; some had also learned nursing procedures needed at home, for example nasogastric feeding, and would do them in hospital as well.

There was a hospital school with two teachers, catering mainly for children of primary school age. The classrooms were not accessible to unaccompanied children, being beyond the double doors which formed the entrance to the ward (Figure 2.1). The school also looked after the occasional older child, probably with work from his own school. Out of school hours and for the younger ones, there was a playleader. There was very little play space, and she had little opportunity to develop her work beyond pastime and occupation. C8 was fairly spacious and the playleader's activities were usually based there. Her constant availability, and the fact that giving attention to those who wanted it was central to her work, made her presence very valuable during the working week.

Observations of the children, and the adults they were with, were made in the 8-bedder, the main corridor outside it, the adjoining corridor and the small playroom which opened off it (see Figure 2.1). They were taken from approximately 6.15 a.m. to 11.30 p.m. The subjects' presence elsewhere was recorded opportunistically, particularly if they were in the corridor outside the unit, where smoking was then permitted. Visitors often congregated there and took children with them, thus frustrating the purpose of the smoking ban within the ward. Observations were not made in the classrooms, or in the bathrooms or toilets, as this would have been too disruptive or intrusive. If

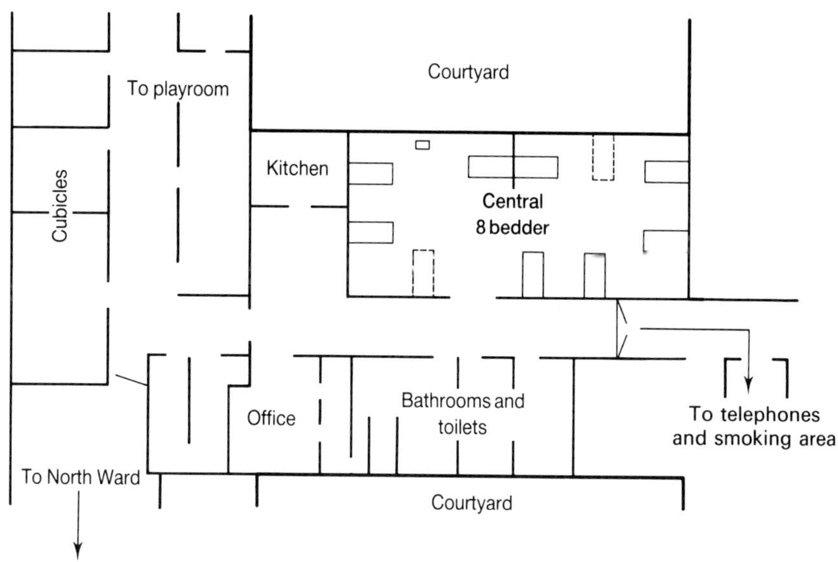

Figure 2.1 Part of Central Ward-C8

children were known to be at school or had been seen in, for example, the office, this was recorded.

The Central Ward 8-bedder was a busy section of the paediatric unit, which received direct, emergency and planned admissions, as well as transfers from cubicles in the same ward, other wards in the unit and other parts of the hospital. In all, 19 children spent some time as patients in C8 during the week of recording, with 12 admissions or transfers to it and 13 discharges or transfers from it; Saturday was the only day when there was no change in the patient population. Only one child was present throughout the week, two others for $6\frac{1}{2}$ days, eight for 2 days or less, and the remaining eight for 3, 4 or 5 days. Nurses will not be surprised to learn that C8 often held nine or 10 beds. Table 2.1 (p.22) gives some general information about the children on the ward during activity sampling.

During the week of activity sampling, the observations provide a series of 'snapshots' of all the occupants of the room, as described at the end of Chapter 1 (and details are given in the Appendix), rather than continuous records of the actions of individuals. Each recording of a child or adult is called a 'sighting' and something happening between two or more people a 'contact'. Percentages given of observations are percentages of sightings, unless something else is specified.

The children in C8 were older than those in North Ward, whose lives are discussed in Chapter 4, having a mean age of 7 years rather than 7 months, so they spent far less of their time asleep – about 20% of the observations compared with 50% of the infants.

Table 2.1 Children admitted to C8

		Age (years)	Length of stay (days)
	n	Range	Range
Males	9	3.9–11.9	2–35
Females	10	1.0–10.9	1–34
Mean		6.9	9.5
Standard deviation		3.9	10.2

The children on the ward who are mentioned by name (these names are, of course, pseudonyms) in the text are:

Alex: nearly 4 – asthma
Claire: $2\frac{3}{4}$ – bronchitis
Gary: nearly 12 – post-neurosurgery; parents resident off-ward
Kevin: $1\frac{3}{4}$ – asthma; resident parent
Laura: $3\frac{1}{2}$ – vomiting and pyrexia
Louise: 9 – diabetes: few visitors
Lucy: $5\frac{1}{2}$ – severe metabolic disorder, a veteran patient
Michelle: 9 – Respiratory tract infection and multiple congenital handicaps
Nicholas: $7\frac{3}{4}$ – blood disorder; resident parent
Paul: 4 – cystic fibrosis, another veteran
Sarah: 10 – cardiovascular disorder
Stacey P: nearly 1 – failure to thrive
Stacey D: 2 – eczema; resident parent or grandparent
Wilfred: 10 – investigations; from cubicle, resident parent

WHERE CHILDREN SPENT THEIR TIME

The age of the C8 patients meant that they were mobile. Only the youngest child (Stacey P) and a severely handicapped girl were not walking independently, although some were restrained for long or short periods by intravenous infusions or monitors. The children were recorded in their beds awake for 28% of observations, in addition to the 20% asleep, but were up and about within the room for rather more than this. The most likely place for a child to be was close to his or her own bed, the area which (the 'bed space') could be enclosed by the curtains; this accounted for about half of the out-of-bed, in-the-room observations. Nearly half of the remainder were seen near the television set, although the children were not necessarily watching television; on the other hand, it was possible to see the screen from about half the beds in C8. The rest of the observations were divided equally between

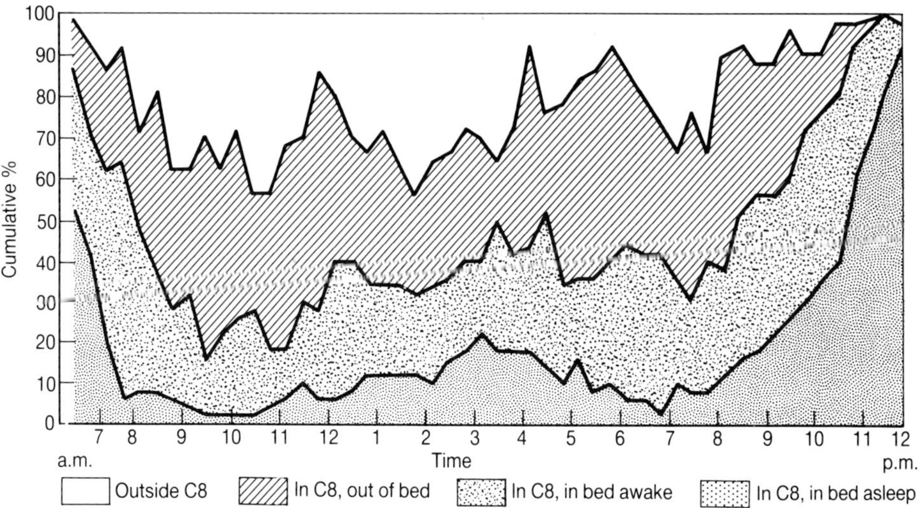

Figure 2.2 C8 patients: in or out of bed, in or out of room; cumulative percentage for each observation point, mean for one week

being in someone else's bed space and in the open area in the middle of the room.

Figure 2.2 shows where children spent their time as a daily pattern, and it is striking that the children were seldom all asleep. All the patients were in bed and asleep at only eight of the 35 observations which were made between 10 and 11.30 p.m.; only the last recording of the day, at around 11.30 p.m., showed nearly all of them asleep. This may have been normal behaviour for some children, while others may have been affected by their individual condition. One boy (Gary) recovering from brain surgery seemed particularly restless and spent 60% of his time away from his own bed space, a third of it outside the room.

Illness, combined with unfamiliar surroundings, the strange requirements of diagnosis and treatment and the absence of familiar night-time rituals, might easily disturb children's sleep. Thus a 2-year-old girl (Stacey D) with eczema went to sleep before 8 p.m. on only one of the six nights she spent in the ward, the other times being between 9.15 and 11.20 p.m., and she would generally refuse to settle except in a pushchair rather than the bed. A 5-year-old (Lucy) who had to go on to intravenous therapy did not go to sleep as early subsequently, and on two occasions was still awake at 11.30 p.m. A boy of 1 year and 9 months (Kevin) was 'settled' for the night at about 7 p.m., but on two of three nights he was to be found up and about again between 8 and 10 p.m. New admissions to the ward late at night did not appear to disturb children nearby unless their beds had to be moved.

When the children were away from C8, they might be seen in other parts of the unit or nearby or, obviously, be quite out of sight. They might be no further away than the bathroom, toilet or the classrooms, where their voices might be heard:

7.40 a.m. SEN (at toilet door) says, 'What are you doing in there?' Paul replies with 'Sitting on the floor.' (Diary 10.10)

8.20 a.m. Bathroom door open. Lucy, Sarah and Andrew are watching nurse (not otherwise specified) bathing Claire; they are all talking. (Record 4.10)

Once Gary was discovered asleep in the linen room, and occasionally older children would retire there to hide from staff (or researchers). They could be further afield for clinical purposes, on an expedition to the shops in the concourse or out for a walk with their parents. Longer-staying patients sometimes went home for a meal or a weekend.

Activity in the corridor

Outside C8, the most common place for children to be was the main corridor immediately outside the room. It was wide and, as Figure 2.1 above shows, joined the corridor where the cubicles and the playroom were at one end, and was closed by double doors at the other. The playroom was very small and was more of a storeroom for larger pieces of equipment than a play area; however, it was freely accessible to patients and their visitors. A broad space branching off the corridor led to the kitchen, while the main arm ran alongside C8 and ultimately out of the unit. The bathroom, toilets and the rather cramped office all opened off the opposite side.

Although it was a corridor, it was not a simple passageway but was, in some ways, the core of the ward. Chairs and a small table there were sometimes used for play or reading stories, and it was wide enough for mobile toys. People, including new patients and ward attenders, might wait or see a doctor in the corridor (there was an X-ray viewer on the wall), and admission procedures sometimes took place there. More importantly, since it provided a vantage point for looking into C8, seeing who was in the corridor itself and, with a few steps, looking down the other corridor, much of the business of the ward went on there. Sisters would direct their staff, teaching rounds held discussions and meals were handed out from the big trolley. Children being assembled for school by the teachers from both South and Central Wards passed that way en route to the classrooms. It served as a promenade for patients and their visitors, and children awaiting visitors would sometimes linger there in order to catch sight of them as soon as they came through the doors. Nurses were often to be found there and used it as an informal nurses' station at night. Spare beds and other equipment might be given temporary space, particularly near the kitchen.

Given the position of the corridor just outside C8 and that it was the arena for so many activities, as well as being on the way to practically everywhere else, it is not surprising that children were so often seen there – just over 30% of the out-of-room observations. A sequence of observations, taken from Wednesday morning, gives a flavour of life there, with almost the atmosphere of a village street:

8.45 a.m.	Lucy, on way back from bathroom, is having hair dried by mother of a female patient from cubicle who is also present.
9.05 a.m.	Doctor and Sister are talking.
9.25 a.m.	Keith and his mother are walking up and down.
9.45 a.m.	Female teacher with two female and three male patients on way to school.
10.05 a.m.	Doctor, 2 physiotherapists, child patient, adult visitor with child in pushchair.
10.25 a.m.	2 doctors, Sister, 2 cleaners, female patient, a father carrying a small patient.
10.45 a.m.	Doctor, father and male patient.
11.05 a.m.	Claire and her mother, two visiting fathers, doctor and Sister.
11.25 a.m.	Sister, mother and doctor, male visitor, a visiting grandfather, Staff Nurse. (Record 5.10)

By the time the next observation took place the lunch trolley would have arrived.

It must not be imagined that all the activity in the corridor meant that quiet and calm reigned in C8 itself. At 8.45 a.m., in addition to Sarah standing near her bed while the sister and an SEN changed the sheets, Claire was sitting up in bed eating. Michelle was behind drawn curtains, another female patient from a cubicle was watching television, while Gary had arrived in a wheelchair pushed by his father, transferred from elsewhere in the hospital. Stacey P was in a baby walker playing with a patient from a cubicle; Stacey D's grandfather was sitting by her bed – she was somewhere else. A boy, who went home later that morning, was rolling about on a big red plastic barrel from the playroom and two doctors were about their business. People without experience of children's wards tend to imagine neat rows of beds, each with a quiet occupant doing nothing more strenuous than a jigsaw puzzle, but this is not the case, nor would it be considered desirable.

Outside the 8-bedder

Table 2.2 (p.26) shows where the children were seen or were assumed to be, when there was available evidence, when they were out of the 8-bedder.

It will be noted that the playroom was little used, partly because it was too full and too small for much active play, and perhaps also because, to a small child, it was far away from his or her own base in the ward, the bed area. When patients from the 8-bedder spent time in one of the cubicles, it usually reflected socialising between parents rather than initiative from the children. Children often sat in silence while the adults talked, while lonely children sometimes wandered into a cubicle where there was a family group, but all

Table 2.2 Location of patients when outside C8: percentage of total 'absent from C8', n = 636

Direction observations (%)		Indirect evidence (%)	
Main corridor	30.3	School	11.6
Playroom and corridor	7.2	Bathroom/toilet	2.2
Smoking area and telephone	3.0	Clinical purposes	2.2
Patient's cubicle	1.9		
Other	0.9	*Unknown*	40.6

generally remained spectators. Friendship between the children might subsequently develop, as between Gary from C8 and Wilfred from one of the cubicles, a boy of Gary's own age but quiet and immature, having received a very sheltered upbringing – quite the opposite of Gary.

> 1.25 p.m. Paul was in another patient's room on the playroom corridor with Laura and Laura's mother. No interaction was taking place between the children, mothers were chatting. (Diary 9.10)

Children's presence in the smoking area was deplored, since it defeated the object of prohibiting smoking on the wards (including the parents' lounge on North Ward), but they were more often there than in the playroom. The area was close to an outside door and could be cold and draughty compared with the wards. Smoking presented parents, particularly mothers, with a dilemma, since they were reluctant to be parted from their children, even briefly, and their anxiety made it unlikely that they would be able to cut down their smoking. The smoking area has since been replaced by a separate room near the main entrance, but the dilemma remains.

The public telephones were not far from the smoking area and were sometimes used by the children as well as their parents, although they occasionally needed help to reach the dials.

Location 'unknown'

When direct observation was impossible, there was obviously underestimation of numbers present, which is reflected in the large proportion of location 'unknown' in Table 2.2 above. The figure for school attendance appears low, but is affected by a variety of factors – only 5% of the 'unknown' relates to children who were available for school. Twelve of the 19 patients during the week were of school age, but three were too ill or arrived too late on Friday to have any opportunity to participate. Two were unable to attend for part of the time because they were receiving intravenous infusions, and another missed a day because of investigation under a general anaesthetic. Sometimes children worked at the bedside rather than in the classroom. Children rarely refused to go to school, like Gary (outside the observation period), but sometimes having gone they returned to the ward because they felt too ill (like Lucy on Wednesday) or were called away for clinical purposes:

> 11.37 a.m. Another doctors' round has arrived, looking for someone in school (Louise is fetched). Twelve people in all (in the round) but she seems undaunted and glad to be out of school. (Diary 10.10)

Taking all these constraints into consideration, school attendance did not account for very much of the 'unknown', even though it is underestimated. The main areas of under-reporting were obviously the use of the bathrooms and toilets and absence for clinical purposes, in the first case, because the children's privacy was respected and, in the second, because only circumstantial or fortuitous evidence was available. Only when a general anaesthetic was involved would the preparations be so obvious or the return to the ward so distinctive that the reason for absence was clear. Absence from the ward for recreational purposes with staff or visitors also falls into this category, since it would only be seen by accident.

LONELINESS AND OTHER PEOPLE'S PARENTS

Whether children are fairly happy while they are in hospital must depend more on whether they are lonely or in reasonably congenial company than on where they spend their time. In the study of babies and small children in an adjoining ward (Cleary 1986 and Chapter 4), the proportion of observations that they spent awake and alone (particularly alone and crying) was used to compare different groups of patients, all of whom were nursed in cubicles. 'Alone' is a much more ill-defined concept within a multibedded room. No child was ever by him or herself in the room during the week, when there were generally six or seven children present, the lowest number being a single observation of three. Adults in the corridor outside the room could see into C8 and were, in some sense, available to the children, just as most of them considered the corridor as part of their territory. Practically no adult would ignore a child in distress or seeking attention, at very least by passing on the message. In the absence of nurses, visitors would help or play with children other than their own or include them with their own families:

> 12.11 p.m. Nicholas's mother went over to talk to and console Stacey P who was crying in high chair. Stacey D and Paul came over to look at [her] and Nicholas's mother drew them into conversation. Nicholas came over and tugged his mother's arm, to go back to his bed space. [His] mother shook her head and said, 'Wait a minute, the little girl is upset.' (Diary 9.10)

> 4.24 p.m. Laura plays in and on her bed with Stacey P.
> 4.25 p.m. Stacey P being bounced up and down by Laura's grandfather.
> 4.55 p.m. Laura and mother, grandmother and grandfather [carrying] Stacey P, all walking towards playroom. (Diary 8.10)

There were 47 occasions (13% of observations) when no nurses were visible in C8 or the corridor (although they were undoubtedly within earshot), and only eight (2%) when there were no visitors – although visitors present at other times were not necessarily those of children in C8. In addition to parents who were resident with their children in the cubicles, three of the observed patients (Stacey D, Nicholas and Kevin) had someone staying overnight with them in the open ward, sleeping on chairs. Two mothers, two fathers and one grandfather (treated as 'parent' in the analysis) were involved. Gary's parents were housed off-ward, and one or both generally stayed in the ward until all the children were asleep. There was no occasion when neither nurse nor visiting adult was present in the room or corridor outside it.

Nevertheless, if a child had no-one near and paying attention, he or she could be considered alone, and almost certainly felt alone in what probably seemed to a small child to be an enormous room. The proportion of observations when these children were recorded 'awake and alone' ranged from 1% to 44%, but these figures include those who were observed only briefly – those discharged on the first day of the study period or admitted on the last. If only the 10 who were recorded over 3 or more days are considered, the three with a parent resident on the ward were classified as 'alone' for less than 5% of observations, Gary for 14%, while for four of the remaining six with visiting parents it was between 20% and 30%. The two exceptions were Laura, aged 3, at 6%, and Paul, aged 4, at 7%. Laura's mother spent practically the whole day on the ward, arriving before 8 a.m. and leaving about 8 p.m., and Laura tended to be miserable when she was not there:

> 12.45 p.m. [Laura] was very unhappy when her mother went to get her own lunch and she was robbed of a toy by Alex's sister. She talked to the observer a little bit, eventually consented to go to the playleader. [She] sat on her lap, then cheered up and played with some toy or other.
> (Diary 7.10)

Paul was in the middle of the rankings for parental visiting (his parents were separated and his father was only recorded on one afternoon), but he received a good deal of professional attention on the ward, particularly from the physiotherapists. He was a veteran patient, very active and sometimes uncooperative, which often resulted in unfavourable staff attention. He frequently sought the company of other patients, their parents and his favourites among the staff:

> 4.35 p.m. Gary and Paul playing chase in playroom corridor.
> 10.15 p.m. Gary's father sitting on floor, playing and talking to Paul, who is sitting on a chair in front of the (switched off) TV set. (Diary 7.10)
> 2.00 p.m. Paul in corridor . . . talking to another (female) patient from a cubicle and in a wheelchair. They both go into C8 to look and see where Paul's bed is. (Diary 8.10)

Occasionally when Paul was seen on a nurse's lap, playing and talking, it was

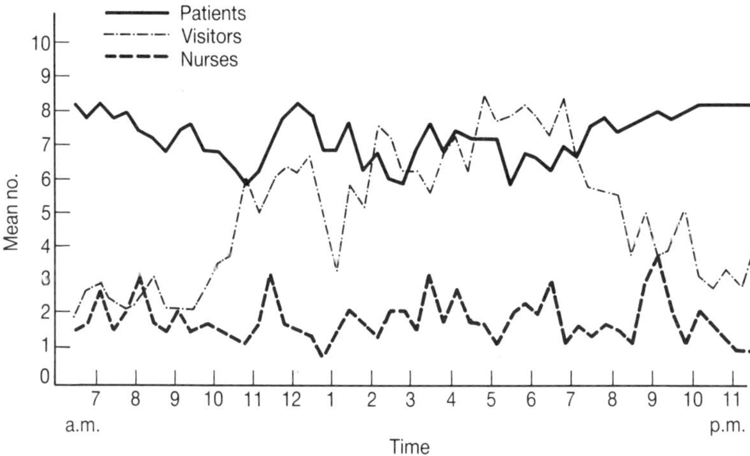

Figure 2.3 Patients, visitors and nurses in C8: mean numbers at each observation point for one week

to ensure that he could be found when impending treatment was due. Sometimes he found himself in a dilemma:

> 9.30 p.m. SEN entered – 'Which one of you is Paul?' Paul is crouching under Gary's bed (presumably hiding, but also) saying 'Nurse, nurse' quite insistently, because one of the nurses [was standing] with her coat on in the doorway and he wanted to say goodbye. (Diary 8.10)

These older children, most of them having language and mobility, were much less likely to show displeasure or distress by crying, although observers sometimes commented on a child looking 'sad' or 'miserable'. The babies on North ward, as a whole, cried for about 20% of 'observed awake', but the children in C8 for less than 2%. Eleven children cried at some time, generally in reaction to some procedure which was being carried out – Paul in particular was inclined to protest when he was put on a drip. Otherwise it was mainly the youngest children, like Stacey P who was very sociable, crying early in the morning when staff were extremely busy and visitors had not begun to arrive.

STAFF, PARENTS AND OTHERS, AND THE TV SET

Figure 2.3 shows the daily pattern of the presence of patients, nurses and visitors in the observed areas, taking the average of the week's observations at each of the 52 recording points in the day. It shows that the presence of nurses echoes the presence of children and has only minor variations throughout the day. Peaks occur at the times of shift change and around mealtimes and, interestingly, in the late evening when nurses might play or chat with the children before they settled for the night:

> 9.50 p.m. The TV was off . . . but nearly all the children [were] wide awake and

the three elder children scampering around. A nursing auxiliary was reading to Lucy, after finishing seeing to her drip, and Paul was listening.

10.10 p.m. Lucy sitting up in bed, close to pupil nurse, who is reading a story. (Record 10.10)

There was no great variation from day to day, particularly if the sightings of nurses are considered in relation to sightings of patients; the ratio of nurses to patients over the week was 0.23. Numbers did not drop at the weekend. The range over the whole day was very similar, the one notably low point being the nurses' lunchtime.

Visitors' presence, not unexpectedly, varied much more during the day. Generally, they began to arrive between 10 and 11 in the morning and left between 7 and 8 in the evening. After that, those who were non-resident were probably staying with children who had been admitted late in the day.

The pattern of visiting did not vary greatly from day to day, except that Sunday, the traditional hospital visiting day, (and to a lesser extent Thursday) showed a short afternoon period of much more intense visiting; there were also a lot of aunts and uncles and other children visiting. The ratio of visitors to patients reached an average of 1.5 between 3 p.m. and 4 p.m. on Sunday. On Thursday there were some grandparents present, and more fathers than usual called in on their way home from work. The mean ratio of visitors to patients for the week was approximately 0.7.

Individual patients might be in contact with a great variety of visitors and staff. They might be with their own mothers, fathers, brothers, sisters, other friends or relations, or with those of another patient, while the staff they met on the ward included nurses (nursing officer, sisters, staff nurses, student nurses, pupil nurses, nursing auxiliaries), doctors (consultants, registrars, house officers) and other professionals (physiotherapists, dietitians, phlebotomists, radiographers). They were also in contact with the playleader, the teachers, the receptionist, medical students, domestic staff and, more occasionally, social workers and chaplains. Each child's pattern of contacts could be very complex, although relatively easy to record when children were in or near their own beds. The interaction categories could be compressed as far as possible to:

own:	parent(s)	nurse(s)
	adult visitor(s)	doctor(s)
	child visitor(s)	other professional(s)
other:	patient(s)	medical student(s)
	parent(s)	others
	adult visitor(s)	playleader
	child visitor(s)	

This produced 60 observed combinations, although only 22 occurred five or more times. Altogether, 1054 contacts at the bed space were recorded: 895

Table 2.3 Patient's contacts at the bed space: summary of 3 groups as a percentage of waking contacts

Contacts with:	%
Parent(s) only	39.6
Parent(s) and any others	29.7
Total parents	66.3
Nurse(s) only	11.5
Nurse(s) and all others	10.2
Total nurses	21.7
Doctor(s) only	1.2
Doctor(s) and others	2.3
Total doctors	3.5

n = total waking contacts at bed space = 895
N.B. Categories including 'others' are not mutually exclusive and cannot be added.

when the child was awake and 159 when asleep. The latter included mothers sitting by their sleeping children as well as nurses attending to intravenous infusions or even giving a nasogastric feed.

From the children's point of view, contacts which take place when they are conscious are obviously of greater importance than those which happen during their sleep. The most frequent contact was with one or both parents, about 40% of those recorded at the bed space (observations of the child awake and in or near his or her own bed comprising more than half the total). This is far greater than any other single type of contact, the next most frequent being with nurse or nurses (at less than 12%), followed by the combination of parent(s) and other adult visitor(s), and then other patients. No other type reaches as much as 5% of contacts. Since categories appear in different combinations, Table 2.3 shows the frequency of contacts with three important groups: parents (including a grandfather), nurses and doctors.

Contacts which included parents and nurses were about 6% of the total, and those with doctors and parents about 2%. Unlike that for the babies in North Ward, personal care generally took place out of sight, and most children were able to attend to their own toileting and feed themselves, thus requiring less attention from nurses. Other patients and their parents were very important as social contacts and sometimes as helpers. Other patients were bed-space contacts for 16% of observations and their parents for 12% (together for only a small proportion of interactions). When children were away from their own beds, their most likely companions were visitors, but this was closely followed by other patients (37.5% and 33.4% of 710 observations respectively).

The playleader worked on the ward for 5 days during the week, and her working time covered 120 observation rounds; for 101 of these she was recorded in contact with children, including children from the cubicles and from North Ward. The children she spent most time with were Lucy, who was largely immobilised by a drip in her foot for most of the week, and Stacey P, the youngest child on the ward, who was undergoing investigations and whose mother was unable to visit as often as she would have liked. The playleader was recorded almost equally in individual bed spaces and elsewhere in the ward.

Overall, the most frequently recorded place to be, away from one's own bed, was by the TV set, although as has been said this did not always mean attending to it – it appeared to be a familiar homely object rather than solely a source of entertainment. Breakfast TV, soap operas and snooker all rolled by, as well as children's programmes. In the evenings, mothers and fathers watched with their children. However, the analysis shows that a third of the recordings of children sitting in front of the television set when it was on (193 in all) refer to one boy – Gary – who would, it seemed, watch anything:

> 9.30 a.m. Most children around TV, only Gary actually watching it – programme about the metabolism of oxygen. (Diary 7.10)

Gary was normally a pupil at a residential school and his viewing there was probably more restricted than most children's.

PLAY AND OTHER PATIENTS

Within the room C8 and away from their own bed space, children were each other's most frequent companions, but the situation for individuals could be quite different. Lucy was confined to bed by a drip, as has been said, but she was a frequent inhabitant of the ward (her mother reckoned that she had had more than 40 admissions in her 5 years), and was familiar with its routines and with the longer-serving staff. She was generally cheerful and sociable and had 'her' bed in the corner near the television set, which tended to be the focus of attention. On Friday, for example, there were 22 recordings of other patients with her, 8 of the playleader, 4 of other mothers and 3 of children from the cubicles. Sarah was twice her age but they spent a lot of time playing and talking together; on the other hand, when Paul, who was only a little younger than Lucy, was near her bed their mothers might be talking but Paul was seldom involved in any interaction.

Some children who were infrequently visited had little social interaction. Louise, aged 9, arrived on the ward on Friday, just before Sarah went home for the weekend, and was on a drip until just about the time Sarah returned to the ward on Sunday evening. Then Louise's life on the ward was transformed. She had been recorded awake and alone for 24 of Saturday's 52 observations, had had about an hour with her own visitors and a period watching television in the evening (the set could not be seen from her bed). Her only other contacts were with nurses and doctors. Sunday was much the same, confined by the drip for most of the day, with visitors at only three observations. When she was liberated, she talked to the other children, but she and Sarah became inseparable, spending every possible moment of Monday in each other's company, generally walking up and down the corridor but joining Sarah's family group when they came in the evening and Louise had no visitors of her own.

The diary record gives examples of the kind of play which children engaged in, with visitors, with staff and with each other. It ranged from general running around and playing about, to more formal games and imaginative play. Reading, even of comics and the like, was rarely mentioned; books other than annuals were hardly ever seen. Gary and Paul, sometimes with Wilfred from one of the cubicles or with Gary's brothers, are described a number of times as 'rushing about', 'playing chase' or 'running in and out of the playroom'. Lucy, too, before she was hampered by the drip set, was seen as running 'all over the place most of the time' (Diary 4.10).

Dolls' prams and pushchairs were popular, sometimes for dolls and sometimes for each other:

10.22 a.m. Stacey D had been laughing and pushing a toy pushchair around . . . with [grandfather] – but cried when he left. (Diary 9.10)

3.36 p.m. Gary and Wilfred pushing each other in the toy baby buggy, quite noisy and excited. (Diary 7.10)

Jigsaws are mentioned a number of times, sometimes as a cooperative activity: Lucy with Gary and a mother from a cubicle, or Lucy with the playleader or Sarah, but Sarah by herself as well. Older children sometimes played board games. While parents played 'pat-a-cake' and 'this little piggy' with the little ones, these children also invented ways of amusing each other. Stacey P's cot was next to Stacey D's bed:

7.50 a.m. Stacey P standing up in her cot, blowing raspberries and Stacey D copying; watching and laughing at each other. When one shook her head repeatedly, the other person mimicked it. Both children found this very entertaining. (Diary 10.10)

Bricks and construction toys of several kinds are mentioned, sometimes for chewing or playful assault rather than their ostensible purpose. Large hollowed-out cubes of red plastic were frequently used – these larger toys gave scope for imagination.

1.55 p.m. There are big play blocks in the playroom, a little like very small armchairs, which can be put together in various ways. Lucy and Sarah had constructed a boat or perhaps a train out of them in the playroom. It seems to me that they were pulling back and forth so I thought it

> was a boat, but Lucy's mother thought it was a train. They put toys in it also, as though they were passengers. (Diary 5.10)

Play was not used systematically to prepare children for procedures or to explore their feelings about their illnesses, nor was there much in the way of 'hospital' play.

The fortunate few who had a resident parent or all-day visitors had scarcely any waking time alone and had someone who could help them break the ice with other children. The younger ones were not always able to join in the play of others and just hung about or failed to make themselves acceptable. The veteran Paul did not have Lucy's skill in dealing with the situation:

> 12.45 p.m. Paul in the corridor by the playroom. Standing on a chair, looking into a cubicle where mother and child have dozens of cars on the table, shouting and occasionally knocking the window, saying, 'My car, my car.' They take no notice. (Diary 9.10)

LIFE IN THE WARD

Within the general pattern, the lives of individual children varied considerably, and some of the influential factors were also individual, rather than clinical. Mobility, maturity and language gave a degree of control over what they did and what happened to them, which was not available to the babies on North Ward. Those with such abilities can make their preferences known and choose whom they approach and, within circumscribed limits, where they go. In order to make the most of the available social interaction, to make friends or find play partners, they required either self-assurance, which was rare, or a mediator, most often a parent. The playleader could perform this function during her working hours, but tended to concentrate her attention on those who were immature, immobile and/or lacked visitors, like Stacey P.

These factors (mobility and maturity) also influenced children's relationships with staff. On North Ward, more than half the recorded interactions were basically part of the treatment and care of the babies and young children (although about half of them included a social component). Technical and professional care was only a small part – less than a quarter – the great majority of interactions being for feeding and ordinary personal care. In the 8-bedder, on the other hand, the use of cubicles for the most seriously ill, and the greater maturity and mobility of the children, meant that the pattern was quite different. They could eat almost unaided and carry out their toileting more or less independently and in private. The vast majority of the interactions seen were purely social, and less than 20% some type of care; of this, about half was technical and professional. This ranged from the distribution and supervision of medication, to managing intravenous infusions and monitoring those who were recovering from procedures under general anaesthesia; these children were also the recipients of the observed personal care. Only the youngest or the most handicapped had to be fed routinely, although the veteran Lucy often had nasogastric feeds, sometimes given by her mother. With this exception, practically all the nursing care was carried out by nursing staff, although the parents of children with cystic fibrosis were often involved in their physiotherapy.

Parents promoted interaction between children more frequently here than in the hospitals where an earlier playleader study was carried out (Hall 1977), where patient and visitor tended to stay by the bedside. The child patients here nearly all wore their own day clothes rather than pyjamas and night-dresses, and this may have altered the parents' perspective on what was appropriate behaviour for the children. There was a significant negative correlation between time spent alone and the presence of parents, which was not simply a reflection of their presence. However, social interaction between parents did not always involve their children, who might remain silent onlookers. It was quite possible for children to be lonely even though they were never completely alone, and the nurses not only regarded playing and talking to children as part of their work, they did it.

The spatial divisions of Central Ward were sometimes related to activity in unexpected ways, the corridor serving as a meeting place, work area and play space, while the playroom was rarely used for its ostensible purpose and the linen store could act as a hidey-hole. The television set was an important focus of activity, a great deal of it nothing to do with its presumed main function.

The 'foreign country' of the hospital is a strange mixture of experiences: the child is basically confined to a bedroom, an enormous one in comparison with his own, and a few adjoining areas, none of which resemble his own home or anyone else's. In the ward, he may have a considerable degree of autonomy since it lacks the continuous supervision and control of mother, father and teacher. In other aspects of his life, particularly on the excursions into the huge, unknown labyrinth of the hospital beyond the ward, strange and distasteful things may be done to him and he is virtually powerless. Life is largely conducted in public and open to the view of the other occupants and passers-by, but the child might nevertheless feel quite lonely or miss privacy. The child who is a stranger to hospitals has to learn new routines for the day and relate to people whose functions – taking his blood or pummelling his chest – he does not understand, but who know a lot about him. On the other hand, about two-thirds of the 19 patients who were observed during this study period had chronic conditions, ranging from psoriasis or asthma to serious congenital anomalies and life-threatening diseases, which could require many episodes of in-patient treatment. For these children hospital will be an important part of life, rather than a single event, and reflect altered prospects in every other aspect of their lives.

REFERENCES

Cleary J, Gray OP, Hall DJ, Rowlandson PH, Sainsbury CPQ & Davies MM (1986) Parental involvement in the lives of children in hospital. *Archives of Disease in Childhood*, **61**: 779–87.

Hall DJ (1977) *Social Relations and Innovation: Changing the State of Play in Hospitals*. London: Routledge & Kegan Paul.

Ministry of Health, Central Health Services Council (1959) *The Welfare of Children in Hospital* (the Platt Report). London: Ministry of Health.

FURTHER READING

Anderson P (1985) *Children's Hospital*. New York: Bantam Press.

Hawthorn PJ (1974) *'Nurse – I Want my Mummy!'* London: RCN.

Mercer D & Mercer G (1986) *Children First and Always: a Portrait of Great Ormond St*. London: Macdonald.

3

Setting up the Care-by-Parent Scheme

Relaxation in visiting practice and parents staying overnight with their children were gradually becoming more common in NHS hospitals in Britain during the 1960s. At the same time, a much more radical change was being suggested in the United States, although it could also be regarded as a return to older ways. Care-by-parent was stimulated not only by concerns about the psychosocial care of children within traditional hospitals, by also by a shortage of paediatrically qualified nurses and the high, almost prohibitive, cost of conventional hospitalisation. Among those who had worked or travelled in the Third World, there was a recognition that family members could take on a meaningful role in the care of patients and that this was essential for the home care of children with long-term conditions.

THE CARE-BY-PARENT IDEA

The idea of a 'domiciliary center' for children who did not need conventional care but needed to attend hospital for 'treatments, procedures or evaluation' was the subject of a feasibility study in Indiana in 1960 (Green & Segar 1961). The study concluded that more than half of the in-patient days of 200 children could have been spent in 'domiciliary' care and that the great majority of parents favoured the arrangement, being most popular with the parents of the younger children.

The first parent-care or care-by-parent unit opened in the University of Kentucky in 1966 (James 1972), the next being the Parent Care Pavilion in Indianapolis in 1971. These were followed by others in many parts of the United States and Canada and were the inspiration for the Cardiff Care-by-Parent Scheme. The American experience is discussed by Suzanne Goodband (with Karen Jennings) in Chapter 9.

WHY CARDIFF?

Cardiff became the site of the first British Care-by-Parent Scheme in 1980 when three sets of interests converged: those from nursing, paediatrics and medical sociology.

In the Cardiff Royal Infirmary, great progress had been made in involving parents in the care of their hospitalised children. The Professor of Child Health (until 1969) in the medical school, AG Watkins, had conducted research which destroyed cross-infection as an argument against unrestricted visiting (Watkins & Lewis-Faning 1949). He also supported Freud's (1949) view of the damaging effects of hospitalisation. His successor, Peter Gray (who retired from the Chair in 1989), had worked with him and shared his views. The new paediatric department at the University Hospital of Wales was designed with parents in mind (rather than nurses some might say), with many single cubicles, where parents could stay with their children, and a sitting room, kitchen and bathroom for their use. Thus, the climate for change was right and there were some facilities available for it.

When Mai Davies (now Nursing Officer – Paediatrics) first came to the Infirmary as ward sister, she found that one condition accounted for a much larger part of the work on the children's wards there than elsewhere. This was spina bifida, which had an increased prevalence in South Wales. The children who suffered from it might have one or two stomas or granulating wounds and they required pressure area care and physiotherapy for their limbs. Unless some alternative could be found, they would spend a great deal of their lives in hospital. Accordingly, Mai Davies began to teach (usually) mothers the nursing skills needed by these children. Others who would also benefit from care at home were those with diabetes and haemophilia. A further group would be able to go home, if only for a weekend at first, if someone in the family could learn nasogastric feeding or tracheostomy care.

All this was particularly important to those for whom the hospital was a regional centre, who might be as much as a hundred miles from home. On the other hand, there were many children who lived within a few hundred yards of this old town centre hospital. Their parents popped in and out, at mealtimes and bedtimes; parents were always expected to carry out normal child care, as far as possible, when they were present.

Parents were allowed to stay overnight, with the choice of a chair by the child's bed or a bed for themselves in the nurses' sick bay. With the move to the new hospital and its increased provision for parents, asking them to stay became part of the admission routine for all patients.

The research element in the situation grew out of the earlier work at Swansea (see Chapter 1) and the continuing interest of Margaret Stacey and myself in the lives of children in hospital. Meeting at a conference, the subject was discussed with the late Marion Ferguson, Director of Nursing Studies at the then Bedford College (but who was formerly of Cardiff). It was felt that it was time for a new observational study of visiting and parental involvement. The idea of care-by-parent – familiar in the literature – came up. Margaret Stacey and Marion Ferguson thought that Cardiff and Peter Gray might be interested in trying it out. I wrote a paper on the subject, with a possible research design. This was September 1980. We then learned that Mai Davies had recently returned from Canada, on a travel scholarship, and had visited the Toronto Care-by-Parent Unit. She was impressed by its philosophy, but felt that some parents were taking on tremendous responsibilities, for example after open heart surgery. Peter Gray was also familiar with the idea, particularly with the Vancouver Scheme: he had already been considering and discussing the topic when we raised it with him.

THE FATE OF PLATT

Also in 1980 the Consumers' Association reported that although there had been great improvements, nearly half of the hospitals they surveyed still restricted visiting in some way, and many which allowed parents to stay did not encourage it, assuring them that it was unnecessary or maybe offering only a hard chair. Facilities for families were generally very poor, and boredom was a great problem:

> It seemed to us that parents were a largely untapped resource and could be used in many ways to the benefit of the children, staff and parents themselves.

One third of the hospitals in the sample admitted children to adult wards where their particular needs were not recognised; this was also true of out-patient departments. There was seldom free access to play facilities for all children at all times.

The majority of children still had multiple carers, rather than the less problematic situation, according to parents, of one or two assigned nurses. The length of stay had been reduced but there was little evidence of the kind of integration of hospital and community services that the Child Health Services Committee (1979) had recommended.

SETTING UP THE RESEARCH

All the elements came together in the autumn of 1980 and the first meeting of the interested parties took place one Saturday in November. From the beginning, it was clear that all sides considered that research was essential to the project – would the scheme work under British NHS conditions, without the financial spur which existed in North America? Getting the money to carry out the study was a long and depressing process. The research design called for the employment of observers and an appropriately qualified nurse, as well as my involvement. Earlier attempts to change the role of parents had been frustrated or slowed to a snail's pace because the effect on nurses' working conditions and job satisfaction had not been considered. The new proposal might have been seen as a threat to the profession of nursing. It also called for a new kind of relationship between nurses and the parents on the ward, the latter becoming partners in care rather than being spectators or helpers.

None of the appropriate government bodies were inclined to continue funding work on children in hospitals, even in the tradition which had produced valuable work in the 1960s and 1970s. Some advisors felt that there was nothing new to say about the role of parents, others that the 'time was not right'. Charitable funds considered it too expensive or thought that the government should be doing it.

The research proposal was written and rewritten. In 1982 an application was made to the Leverhulme Trust, who were interested in the idea and felt that they could fund one full-time researcher and the observers necessary to cover the whole of the working day during data collection periods, as well as other support costs. Several more attempts to fund a nursing researcher were made but proved unsuccessful.

In the hospital, a steering committee had been set up, which included representatives from administration, the Health Authority and the Department of Nursing Studies, the Director of Nursing Services and those most involved in the paediatric unit. On the academic side, it was joined by Margaret Stacey, Marion Ferguson and David Hall (now lecturing at the University of Liverpool). One question which had to be dealt with very early on (long before the matter of funding was settled) was that of legal responsibility when unqualified, non-employed people are carrying out nursing work. The hospital's legal advisor gave it as his opinion that there was no problem:

> Provided that the medical and nursing staff of the Paediatric Unit understand that their responsibility is not diminished by involving the parents, any more than it would be diminished by using other helpers who are not fully trained or professionally qualified, then I see no need for any legal problems to arise.

When the Lexington Unit was first set up, parents were described as 'in effect, [filling] the role of auxiliary personnel' (McClure & Ryburn 1969). This view is supported by Dimond (1989).

Permission for the research to take place was received from both the medical and nursing ethics committees.

PLANNING THE SCHEME

Various ideas about the format of the Care-by-Parent Scheme were floated but sank. One was that the six cubicles at one side of North Ward (presently caring for babies and very young children) could be divided off and treated as a unit for all ages. This had to be abandoned because clinical considerations were paramount, and every cubicle, particularly those with piped oxygen, had to be available for seriously ill children. It also proved impossible to accommodate older children in these cubicles because larger beds could not be evacuated from them if the need arose, nor were there children's toilet or bathing facilities on this ward – only baby baths and provision for adults. In the event, the great majority of the participants in the scheme during the data collection period were infants on North Ward, although some were older children on Central Ward. The main surgical ward, which had a smaller proportion of cubicles, did not join in the scheme at this stage.

Work, or rather paid work, on the scheme began early in 1983. Research instruments – recording sheets for observations, coding schemes, questionnaires for nurses and parents – had to be designed and piloted, as did explanatory letters for both staff and parents about the nature and purpose of the research. Observers had to be recruited and trained; the advertisement stressed the awkward hours (early mornings and late nights in a 7-day week), and that it was part-time, temporary and not very well paid, but despite this there was a very good field of applicants. A mix of experience with children in normal situations and familiarity with the hospital environment was required, and this was achieved. There were nine observers in all (in addition to the author who also acted as one) – seven at each stage. Four of them were experienced teachers, two were mature psychology graduates (one of whom was also an SRN), one a graduate nurse, one a physiotherapist and one a nursing auxiliary. Most had children of their own and were hoping to return to full-time work in their own professions. Discussions within the hospital made it clear that the scheme was regarded as an initiative within the paediatric unit, perhaps only for research purposes. As it was not making any demands for extra staff or finance, the unit managers had complete freedom to run the scheme as they wanted, but it also meant that its existence was informal and ran the danger of being ephemeral.

The concept of a 'philosophy of care' was not in use at the time, but the senior staff all had a strong commitment to a style of nursing which included parents, rather than seeing them as peripheral to care.

SELECTION

One question which had to be settled was which children would be suitable for care-by-parent. A statement outlining this, which was drawn up for the Leverhulme Trustees, follows. A shorter version, which included asthma as well as the conditions specified below, was posted up in the ward offices.

> Parent-care for child inpatients, as envisaged in the proposed study, is not intended and could not be appropriate for all such children. Many children in hospital require a high degree of professional expertise and its accompanying technology, if they are to make a successful and speedy recovery. Parent-care is not for them, at any rate until they are nearing the end of their hospital stay.
>
> The principal criterion for a child's admission to the parent-care unit will be the child's medical condition. Three factors are involved in the decision in every case:

1. although medical supervision is necessary the nursing care required is minimal or of the kind that any mother would normally expect to carry out;
2. the likelihood that the condition will recur will be lessened if the family's general health education can be improved, e.g. in matters of diet and hygiene;
3. where the condition is long-term or chronic and specific techniques of observation or treatment must be learnt and carried out at home, if the child is to live at home and the effects of the condition are to be minimised.

Professor Peter Gray has listed conditions treated in his department which he regards as appropriate for parent-care, either by direct admission to the scheme or by transfer to it, when the acute phase of an illness has passed or an operation has been carried out and the child is recovering. Those involving chiefly the first and/or second factors are:

(i) the investigation of failure to thrive or feeding problems in babies or growth problems in older children;
(ii) chest infections, urinary infections and gastro-enteric infections which tend to recur;
(iii) kidney diseases;
(iv) febrile convulsions;

Those in which the third factor is crucial:

(v) diabetes is the commonest member of this group; the parents and the older child need to learn about the regulation of diet, the preparation and giving of injections, as well as the clinical signs that emergency treatment may be required.
(vi) coeliac disease which requires particular attention to diet;
(vii) cystic fibrosis, which requires constant physiotherapy to maintain adequate lung function; medication and attention to diet are also crucial;
(viii) babies who must remain in hospital unless their mother can learn special feeding techniques, like tube-feeding and the management of cleft-palate;
(ix) similarly, the care of children with tracheostomies.

This list was specific to the University Hospital of Wales and therefore did not include conditions normally treated at other hospitals in the district, for example, leukaemia.

The question of suitable parents was frequently raised at meetings of the steering committee and caused some disquiet. Administrators in particular were concerned about possibly irresponsible parents who would not be sufficiently careful in carrying out the observations and procedures they had taken on. The researchers tended to worry that the selection would be over-careful and that only the well-spoken and well-educated would be invited to take part. The nurses, basing their judgement on their experience of parents, had no particular qualms. They considered that parents would select themselves and only those who felt able to take on the responsibility would volunteer to join the scheme – they were, of course, quite right. When the topic was discussed with parents in general terms before the scheme began operating, some, although attracted by the idea, were dubious about their own ability. The question most frequently raised, however, was whether or not the scheme would result in the loss of nursing jobs – if it did, parents said they would disapprove. This reaction was caused, presumably, by the past history and current state of unemployment in South Wales.

THE SCHEME BEGINS

The first phase of the observations, which took place in October 1983, provided information about the lives of children who were being nursed conventionally in a unit which welcomed parents and made use of their abilities. For the majority of children this is the best available solution when in-patient care is necessary. The observations were also intended as a basis for comparison with the later care-by-parent stage; many of the findings are reported in Chapter 3. The second stage of observations, when the Care-by-Parent Scheme began operating, started on May 1st 1984. It had been intended to postpone these observations until the scheme had been working for some time, but it appeared that without the impetus provided by the research presence, the start might be long-delayed, and the research timetable could not accommodate this.

It had been decided that when a child was thought suitable for care-by-parent according to the guidelines (the same criteria used for case study children in the first phase), the parents should be approached by a senior registrar, who would describe the scheme and leave them with a copy of the leaflet about it. They were given a few hours to consider the matter and then a ward sister (usually) would answer their questions and ask whether or not they wished to join the scheme. If they did – and during the study period practically everyone did – the care-by-parent (CBP) nurse would be introduced and the process could begin. Involving a senior registrar proved to be impractical and unnecessary, so, the task was taken over by the ward sisters.

At the beginning of each shift, one of the nursing staff became the 'designated nurse' who was responsible for the Care-by-Parent Scheme while she was on duty. The constant variation in staff meant that only some qualified nurses could build up their expertise. The demands of the case mix at the time determined who would take on the responsibility for that shift. The ideal person for the job was one who was well qualified and mature enough to have the necessary knowledge, appreciative of the practical and emotional difficulties that parents might face, and able to understand the kind of teaching that was required. Within the ward team, the best person for the job was the second most senior: the most senior had too many other responsibilities and could often be called away to attend to something else, perhaps in the middle of supervising a mother carrying out a procedure for the first time.

However, the needs of the very sick children or illness among the staff might mean that learner nurses had to take on the job. Their natural teaching skills and self-confidence varied and there was no opportunity for specific training. Some were inclined to slip in and do something themselves when the parents were absent for a few minutes. An observer heard an auxiliary nurse berating a student who was the CBP nurse at the time: 'Why are you doing that when there is a bloody great teddy bear stuck up outside?' (a teddy bear was the symbol which indicated that a patient was involved in care-by-parent). The observer also saw that the mother was on her way back to the cubicle. The student nurse may have done this simply because it was quicker for her to do whatever was needed, but there were also difficulties in reaching a common knowledge base. On one occasion a nurse (unqualified) described how she and a mother had found the baby's radial pulses and each had held it for the requisite time. At the end she discovered that the mother had not counted the rate and felt that this indicated a lack of sense in the mother and inherent weakness in the whole idea. An outsider might think it meant that the nurse had assumed too much or had not effectively explained what was wanted. Even adults are usually told about their pulse rate in general rather than numerical terms. The mother may have been attempting to assess the rhythm and strength of the beat, or, perhaps, at that point finding and keeping track of the pulse was as much as could be expected of her. Nurse and mother were at cross purposes, and the episode probably lowered the mother's confidence in her ability.

It was often difficult for nurses to comprehend just how little a mother or father might know about the nature and purpose of what was going on or could recall in a time of stress. The school-leaver who wants to be a nurse has a specific knowledge and interest which the intending lawyer or shop assistant does not share – and mothers in both of these occupations took part in the scheme. The development of leaflets for parents on carrying out common procedures (described in Chapter 7) meant that staff learned to spell out the components of each process in great detail, but this did not take place until much later on.

The CBP nurse had all the care-by-parent children as his or her assigned patients; if children were numerous (six was the largest number observed at any one time) or they all required the maximum input of nursing time, a second nurse might be associated. If there were very few children, the CBP nurse would have other assigned patients as well. The nurse wore a badge with a picture on it, a larger version of which was attached to the cubicle doorpost, so both nurse and patient could be easily identified. Initially, a red teddy bear was used, but then a panda was adopted because black and white was easier to reproduce; recently the CAPS (Cardiff Assisting Parents Scheme) logo has been used.

When a parent had agreed to join the scheme, the CBP nurse was introduced and the teaching process could begin. In the early days, and certainly during the research period, teaching usually began with the measurement of temperature, pulse and respiration: first watching it being done, then learning how to record it, next carrying it out under supervision and finally doing and recording it solo. Originally, taking the vital signs was taught to everyone, because they were part of every child's routine and seemed simple to the staff. Also, since they were taken several times a day, there were many opportunities for practice. Experience has shown that this is not the best way to start and parents now usually begin with something simpler, such as the fluid balance chart.

Changes have also taken place in the way the scheme is run on the wards – the major alteration is described in Chapter 7. However, after the research and several changes at ward sister level, there was a move away from the idea of a designated CBP nurse responsible for all the children. Instead, children were assigned like the other patients, so that one nurse could have several conventionally-nursed and one CBP patient in her charge. This may have had advantages in terms of workload and skill mix but tended to dilute the nurses' experience of the scheme and, to some extent, dissipated its strength.

CARE-BY-PARENT PATIENTS AND PARENTS

In practice, in both the research period and since, the majority of children in the scheme have been babies on North Ward. The accommodation there is in cubicles and there are more resident parents who can be candidates for care-by-parent. Consequently, a degree of expertise in managing care-by-parent grew up there and was more readily available. The fact that in a babies' ward a very large part of nursing time is spent in personal care, like bathing, toileting and feeding, also made it a more obviously feasible option from the staff point of view. Mothers' perceptions of the helplessness of babies and their heightened awareness of their needs – what Robertson and Robertson (1982) call 'an irresistible commitment to the baby's wellbeing' – makes it easier for them to overcome their feelings of diffidence and incompetence when faced with professionals on their own ground. They are more likely to continue or resume care of their babies in hospital than of their older children, unless the latter are disadvantaged by physical or mental handicap or chronic illness. The more complex, less obvious, psychosocial needs of the pre-school and school-age child are still less well understood, despite decades of evidence.

During the 5 weeks of observations after the CBP scheme had begun, 72 children were patients in North Ward, five of whom were admitted twice (only one for a different reason). Forty-four of them had a resident parent, of whom 27 joined the scheme. At the first stage, there were 78 patients in the ward – three admitted more than once and 37 with a resident relative. These differences are not statistically significant ($Chi^2 = 2.295$). The resident relatives for both periods were mainly mothers, but some fathers took over or shared care, as did a few grandmothers and the occasional grandfather or aunt.

In both study periods nearly half the admissions were for respiratory and gastroenteral infections. The next largest group was of children with serious conditions, like central nervous system and severe metabolic disorders, whose lives were punctuated by hospital admissions. These two groups overlapped somewhat, since a minor infection would be more likely to result in hospitalisation for a child with grave underlying problems than it would an otherwise healthy child. This is also true of those with congenital heart conditions, but they were more often seen pre- and post-cardiac surgery performed elsewhere. Another large group was of children admitted for investigations, most often described initially as 'failure to thrive' or '? fitting'. Other infections and skin conditions formed the majority of the rest.

Each of these groups could provide candidates for care-by-parent. The basic assumption of the system is that almost any child will benefit from being looked after by familiar people rather than strangers, however skilled they may be. If this is now accepted (and in the past it was not), the question remains of how far it is feasible and safe, given that hospitalisation implies the need for something more specialised than ordinary home care. Among the patients' families, there were many who could learn the nursing skills necessary to look after children with transient infections, once any danger had passed, and who would profit from the general health education it often involved. Children with long-term conditions would be able to spend more time at home the more skilled their parents became. Being part of the care-giving process throughout their stay provides parents with the best opportunity to develop competence and confidence. They also learn to observe and make appropriate decisions about seeking professional advice or care. Children who are undergoing investigations need mainly routine care, reassurance and distraction (particularly if the tests involve discomfort or fasting), which parents should be able to provide.

Care-by-parent also provides opportunities for staff to observe the way the child is handled and treated, which may be relevant to the diagnosis. Some of these children, sadly, will join the frequently admitted, the 'veterans', and while the parents' experience will be stressful, involvement may provide a less traumatic introduction to the wards and the staff they will get to know well in the future.

The management of the CBP Scheme has remained within the control of the nurse managers of the paediatric unit. In 1988 an addition to the staff was provided in the form of a sister, without ward responsibilities, who would manage the scheme, which now operated on all three wards. Her unforeseen but unavoidable departure, which more or less coincided with the retirement of Peter Gray, has provided, if nothing else, an opportunity to reassess the working of the scheme and the best way to ensure its successful operation and secure its future.

REFERENCES

Child Health Services Committee (1976) *Fit for the Future* (the Court Report). London: DHSS, DES and Welsh Office.

Consumers' Association (1980) *Children in Hospital: A Which? Report*. London: Consumers' Association.

Dimond B (1989) Legal aspects of paediatric nursing. *Nursing Times*, **85**: 70–1.

Freud A (1949) Children in hospital. *Lancet*, **i**: 784–6.

Green M & Segar WE (1961). A new design for patient care and pediatric education in a children's hospital: an interim report. *Paediatrics*, **28**: 825–37.

James VL (1972) Care by Parent unit cuts costs, benefits hospitalized child. *Hospital Topics*, **50**: 72–4.

McClure MJ & Ryburn AC (1969) Care-by-Parent unit. *American Journal of Nursing*, **69**: 2148–52.

Robertson J & Robertson J (1982) *A Baby in the Family: Loving and Being Loved.* Harmondsworth: Penguin.

Watkins A & Lewis-Faning E (1949). Incidence of cross-infection in children's wards. *British Medical Journal*, (2): 616–19.

FURTHER READING

Azarnoff P & Hardgrove C (eds.) (1981) *The Family in Child Health Care*. Chichester: John Wiley and Sons.

Bivalec LM & Berkman J (1976) Care-by-parent – a new trend. *Nursing Clinics of North America*, **11**: 109–13.

Caldwell B & Lockhart LH (1981) A care-by-parent unit: its planning, implementation and patient satisfaction. *Children's Health Care*, **10**: 4–7.

Green M & Green JG (1977) The parent-care pavilion. *Children Today*, **6**: 5-8, 36.

James VL & Wheeler WE (1969) The care-by-parent unit. *Paediatrics*, **43**: 488–94.

Lerner MJ, Haley JV, Hall DS & McVarish D (1972) Hospital care-by-parent: an evaluative look. *Medical Care*, **X**: 430–6.

Robinson GC & Clarke HF (eds.) (1980) *The Hospital Care of Children: a Review of Contemporary Issues*. New York: Oxford University Press.

Tonkin P (1979) Parent care for the low risk and terminally ill child. *Dimensions in Health Service*, **56**: 42–3.

Vermilion BD, Ballantine TVN & Grosfeld JL (1979) The effective use of the parent care unit for infants on the surgical service. *Journal of Pediatric Surgery*, **14**: 321–24.

4

Care-by-Parent Begins: Life in Three Care Groups

OBSERVATIONS IN NORTH WARD

During the activity sampling observations on North Ward (Figure 4.1, p.50), there were 26 child patients, of whom 10 – the NRP group – were without a resident parent. Seven children – the RP group – had a parent resident but were not in the CBP scheme (one was transferred to CBP, but was then discharged within hours), and nine – the CBP group – were nursed in the Care-by-Parent Scheme. On average during the week, there were 12 patients in the ward, with a range of 9–14, representing a bed occupancy rate of about 86%. During the following 4 weeks of observation, bed occupancy was slightly higher – nearly 90%; on three nights there were 15 patients in the 14 cubicles. The analysis of the activity sampling data allows the reader to compare the lives of children in three situations, but in the same place, at the same time and with the same group of staff.

Observational research within hospital wards has particular problems, especially that it is impossible to produce a neat experimental situation, with index and control subjects nicely matched. Variables cannot be controlled since the patients' sex, age and condition all change at random. Even when the same child is present for comparison on two occasions, he or she is older and wiser in the ways of the hospital and the illness (or more disturbed by them) on the second admission. There are staff changes, too, which obey another set of rules, while a different time of year may bring a different case mix and variations in the pattern of behaviour – summertime may mean more trips outside and more wakeful evenings.

It would have been possible to compare life on North Ward in May, when the Care-by-Parent Scheme began, with life on North Ward in the previous autumn, when the initial observations were made: a 'before and after' comparison. The case mix was similar, but any differences which emerged from the analysis might have been due to other factors. There were changes in the

Table 4.1 Patients present during activity sampling: May 1984, North Ward

	NRP (n = 10)	RP (n = 7)	CBP (n = 9)
Age in weeks:			
Range	3–107	0.3–48	3–89
Mean	29.7	24.8	36.6
Length of stay in days:			
Range	4–119	1–9	2–7
Mean	29.6	3.6	4.0

nursing personnel and the learners had begun to do their paediatric work at a different stage of their course. The time of year affects people's behaviour, but perhaps more importantly, so does the particular combination of staff, children and families and the way they interact with each other. Concentrating on three groups separated by a factor of paramount interest, the degree to which parents were involved in their children's lives on the ward, but who were present at the same time has the advantage of reducing other variations which could have affected the results.

It will be seen from the data in Table 4.1 that the chief difference between the groups is that the NRP group had a much longer mean length of stay. This was due partly to the presence of three children with very long admissions. They all suffered from congenital abnormalities and one, with a stay of 119 days, was the subject of legal proceedings which delayed both treatment and discharge. A long stay is not in itself a barrier to CBP, and increasing the parents' nursing skills will shorten it. In the following year, one mother stayed in hospital with her son, who had a malabsorption syndrome, for 4 months, originally having been in another hospital. In Cardiff she joined the CBP Scheme and was able to take her baby home after she had learned to manage total parenteral nutrition.

Children in the RP group had a somewhat narrower age range than the other two groups.

LIFE IN THE WARD

The following children are mentioned by name in the text. All were patients in North Ward unless otherwise stated, and those whose names are underlined are those nursed in the CBP Scheme.

Andrew: 3 weeks/8 months – flocculent hydrocephalus, see case study below

Brian: 1 – Respiratory tract infection; Central Ward; mother in hospital for surgery

Craig: 3 months – investigations

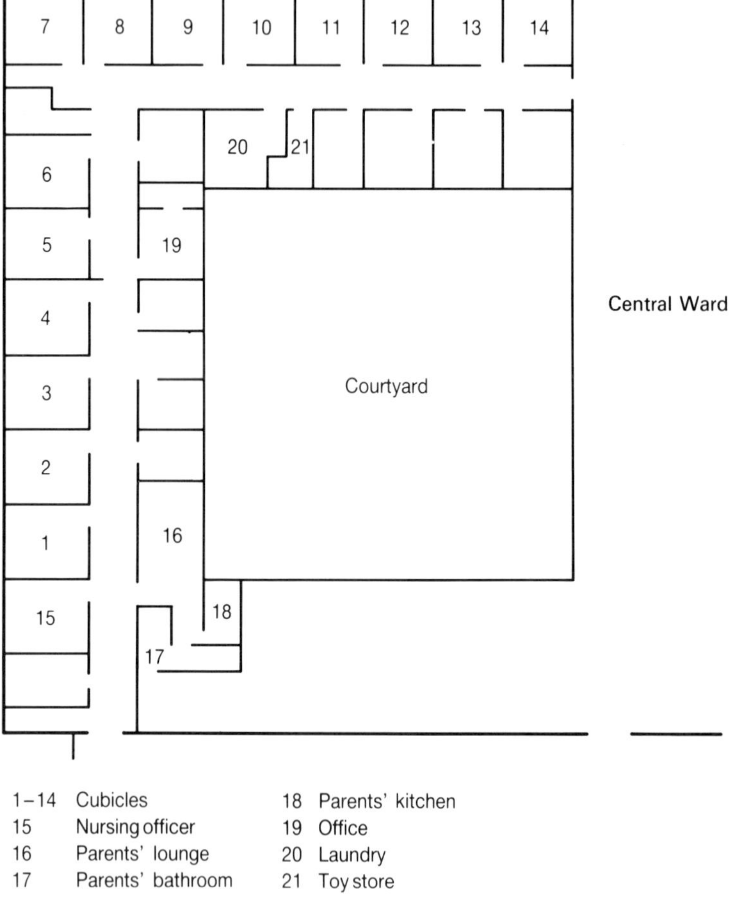

1–14	Cubicles	18	Parents' kitchen
15	Nursing officer	19	Office
16	Parents' lounge	20	Laundry
17	Parents' bathroom	21	Toy store

Figure 4.1 North Ward ground plan

Emma: 10 months – Upper respiratory tract infection; Central Ward
Jyoti: 10 months – pneumonia, a twin
Kenneth: 1 year/1 year 7 months – Lower respiratory tract infection, multiple congenital handicaps, see case study below; Central Ward
Maria: 12 – severely handicapped following illness; Central Ward
Lucy: 6 – severe metabolic disorder, a 'veteran'; Central Ward
Paul: $4\frac{1}{2}$ – cystic fibrosis, another 'veteran'; Central Ward
Peter: $1\frac{1}{2}$ – facial oedema, allergy
Sarah: 1 year 4 months – investigations, including jejunal biopsy
Sean: 2 months – recurrent apnoea
Simon: 1 year 10 months – congenital hydrocephalus

Each of the three groups of children included some with gastroenteritis,

Table 4.2 Three care groups: alone or with someone, asleep or awake: % of total observations

	NRP	RP	CBP
Asleep:			
Alone	49.7	16.9	24.1
With someone	5.1	23.1	22.9
Total asleep	54.9	40.0	47.0
Awake:			
Alone	19.8	9.4	3.4
With someone	25.3	50.6	49.6
Total awake	45.1	60.0	53.0
Total alone	69.5	26.3	27.5
Total with someone	30.5	73.7	72.5
Total observations (n)	2684	563	978

some with chest infections and others with feeding difficulties or poor weight gain, which might be physical in origin or a problem of management. There were two children with hydrocephalus in the NRP group and one in the RP group during activity sampling; later there were three in the CBP group and Andrew is the subject of a case study (see below). Table 4.2 and Figure 4.2 (below) give the bare bones of life in the ward for the three groups: asleep or awake, alone or with someone (who is sometimes referred to as a 'contact').

The total number of observations for the NRP group is larger than for either of the others, not only because they were a slightly larger group, but also because they had on average longer stays, and those who were the least visited rarely left their cubicles or the corridor outside it. They were, therefore, always there to be recorded. All but one (who had the shortest stay) were alone for more than 60% of observations. In the RP group, only one was alone for more than 50% of observations, and two for less than 10%. Among the CBP children, four were alone for less than 20% and five for between 25% and 42% of observations.

Children in the NRP group, despite including the oldest children, slept more than those in either of the other groups, which the paediatricians regarded as developmentally undesirable, particularly as they tended to stay in hospital longer than the others. Even without the three exceptionally long stays (60–119 days), the mean stay for this group was 6.7 days. They also spent much more of their time alone. Certainly, a large proportion of this was when they were asleep – or perhaps they were asleep because they were alone and their environment was lacking in stimulation. Being alone does not matter to sleeping children, but it probably means that they are alone when they are going to sleep and alone when they wake up, which is very different from the situation of the sick child at home. There were great differences within the NRP group as well: they ranged from children who had a parent with them from breakfast time until late evening (the observations covered the period from about 6.15 a.m. to 11.30 p.m.), even when this meant occupying another child as well, to a few who were scarcely visited at all. One, a baby with a serious congenital heart condition, lived 60 miles away, while another lived locally but was only visited for about $2\frac{1}{2}$ hours during the 6 days he was observed, about half the length of his stay.

When the figures for the other two groups, both with resident parents, are examined it transpires that those who were in the RP group were awake and alone more than two and a half times as often as those in CBP (RP 9.4%, CBP 3.4%). It seems possible that those who were not involved in the nursing care of their children felt inadequate in comparison with the professionals and unable to meet their children's needs, so found it less painful or less frustrating to be somewhere else.

Crying

Figure 4.2 compares the three groups of children, whether asleep or awake, alone or with someone. The squares represent all the observations of the particular group of children and the individual elements percentages of them. They show how the NRP children were more often alone than either of the other groups, and that the RP children were awake and alone more than the CBP group. The figures also represent the amount of crying that went on. Since the children in North Ward were nearly all babies, crying is a definite indication of unhappiness or some unmet need, whether for food, company, comfort or relief from pain or discomfort. Babies have only one means of drawing attention to their needs, which has the advantage for observers of being easily identifiable – except for the children with tracheostomies, of whom there was one among the case studies. If babies are crying and with someone, they stand a good chance of having their needs met. Although the crying may have been caused by a disturbing or uncomfortable procedure – taking blood or simply changing a nappy. Crying occupies quite a large part of the waking time of all of the patients, but the proportions vary among the three groups. Most of the difference is accounted for by 'crying alone' for which the figures are NRP 10.7%, RP 4.4%, CBP 2.1%.

Children without a resident parent who were being barrier nursed were at a particular disadvantage because going to see what they wanted could not be done incidentally, fitting it in with other work. Those who were at the far end of the ward, like Craig, were also unlucky, because they were a long way

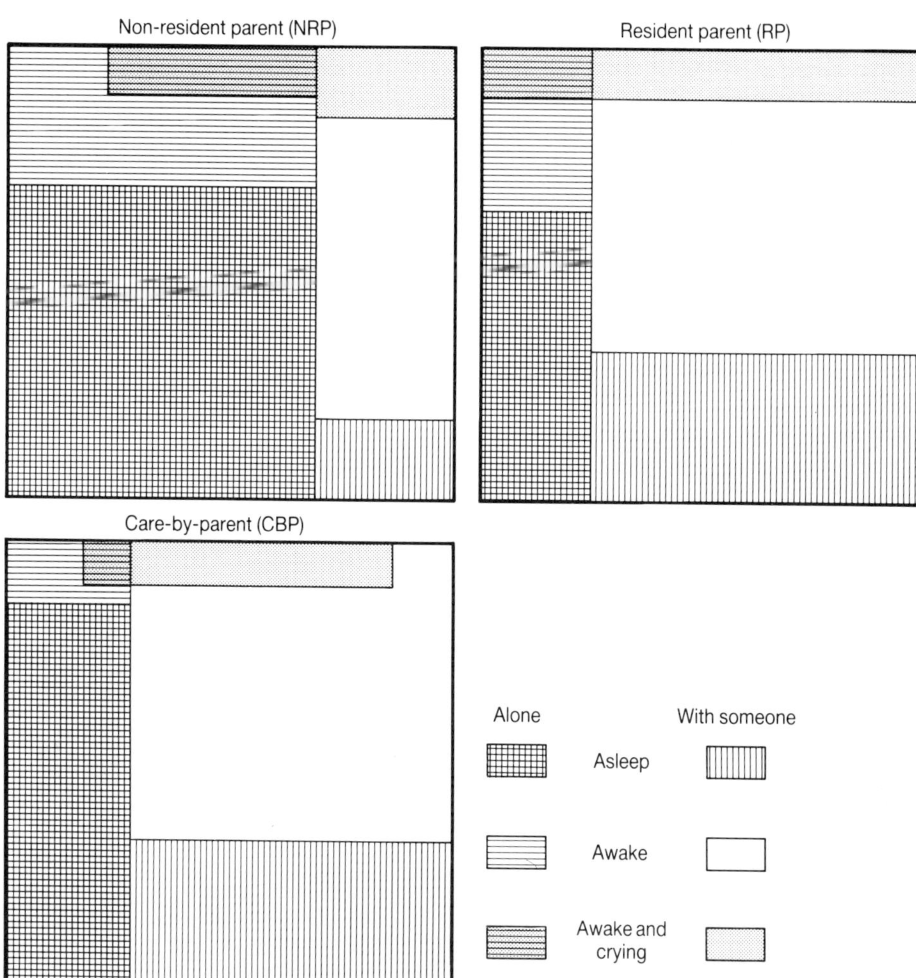

Figure 4.2 Pattern of life: three care groups compared: percentage of total observations

from the centre of activity and there were few passers-by to distract them. Craig was in cubicle 14 and was recorded crying for 38.2% of 'awake', two-thirds of it when he was 'alone'. One of the aims of modern practice is to cut down the number of people handling any one child, but feeling ignored may prove more damaging. A few children, inconsolable in the absence of their mothers when no amount of attention could comfort them, eventually cried themselves to sleep. Strangely, one of the CBP children scarcely stopped crying, although her mother was there and attentive. Jyoti was about 10 months old and was one of the case study children:

11.15 a.m. Jyoti crying continuously, mother very worried, looks exhausted.

> Tried to distract her with toys, talking, cuddling, rocking in pram – little success. (Diary 17.5)

Jyoti was recorded crying for 45% of her time awake, but was only alone for 10 seconds of this. She was a twin and, although her sister visited, it seems likely that separation from her was the disturbing factor. Therefore, as soon as her condition had been diagnosed and treatment established, she was discharged. With the baby so upset and a total stay of less than 48 hours, her teacher mother had little opportunity to learn any nursing skills, although she was keen to do so.

Who children spent their time with

Unlike on the 8-bedder open ward, it was fairly easy to decide whether a child was alone or with someone and, because of their age, children either could not move independently or would not be allowed to do so unaccompanied. When they were with someone they might be with family members – mothers, fathers, grandparents, brothers and sisters were frequent visitors to the ward – with staff, or with a combination of the two. Figure 4.3 shows not only what proportion of the time someone was with them, both sleeping and waking, but which group of possible contacts they fell into.

The NRP children were with staff twice as often as they were with family members, and 'staff' means a very much larger number of people than the most extended family. There was very little overlap between staff and the family, so they had very little opportunity for exchanging information or getting advice. The RP and CBP groups more or less reversed the NRP figures, being with their families about as much as the NRP were alone. The RP group were in contact with the staff more than those in CBP, but staff were combined with the family much more than in the NRP group. The CBP children were seldom with staff only, this usually when nurses took over while a mother had a break, or sometimes when they took advantage of her absence to check the charts. This was a pity because most mothers enjoyed the interest, reassurance or extra instruction if the check was made while they were there.

THE NATURE OF CARE AND INTERACTION

Having a mother or father present provides the child with what Bowlby (1988) calls 'a secure base', which is most important when the child is 'frightened, fatigued or sick'. The need then 'is assuaged by comforting and care-giving', which is more active than simply being there. The kinds of interaction that went on are displayed in Figure 4.4 (p.56): feeding and personal care, nursing and medical care, and filling social needs by talk, play and comforting. In Figure 4.4 the squares represent the total of interactions, not observations as in the previous two sets of data. Interactions are a

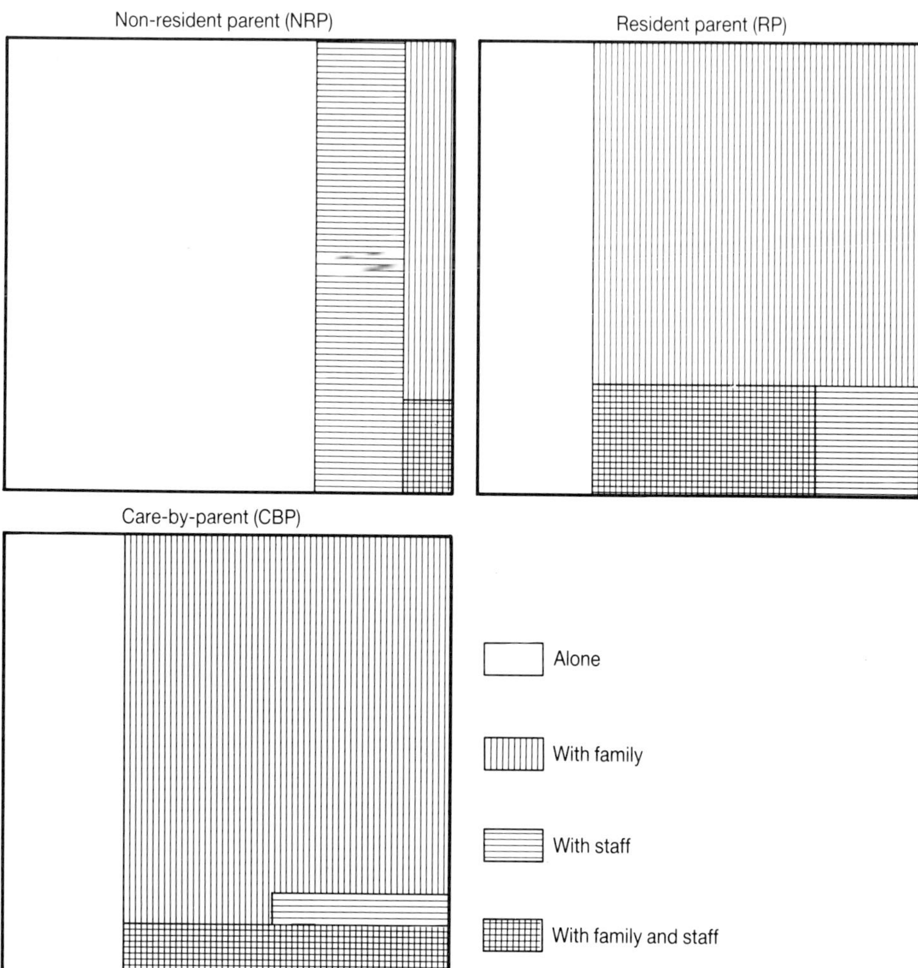

Figure 4.3 Nature of contacts: three care groups compared: percentage of total observations

proportion of contacts – Table 4.3 (p.56) and the shaded areas in Figure 4.3 above show how they both relate to total observations for the three care groups. If the NRP group's interactions were shown in proportion to those of the other groups, the square would be about half the size.

For the NRP children, interactions formed a very high proportion of contacts, which reflects the amount of time they spent alone. The person with them was most often a member of the hospital staff, generally for a specific purpose (Cleary 1979). The pictures for the two groups with resident parents are very similar.

More of the NRP children's interactions are to do with feeding and

Table 4.3 Contacts and interactions: % of observations

	NRP	RP	CBP
Contacts (%)	30.4	73.7	72.5
Interactions (%)	22.5	41.7	42.0
Observations (n)	2684	563	978

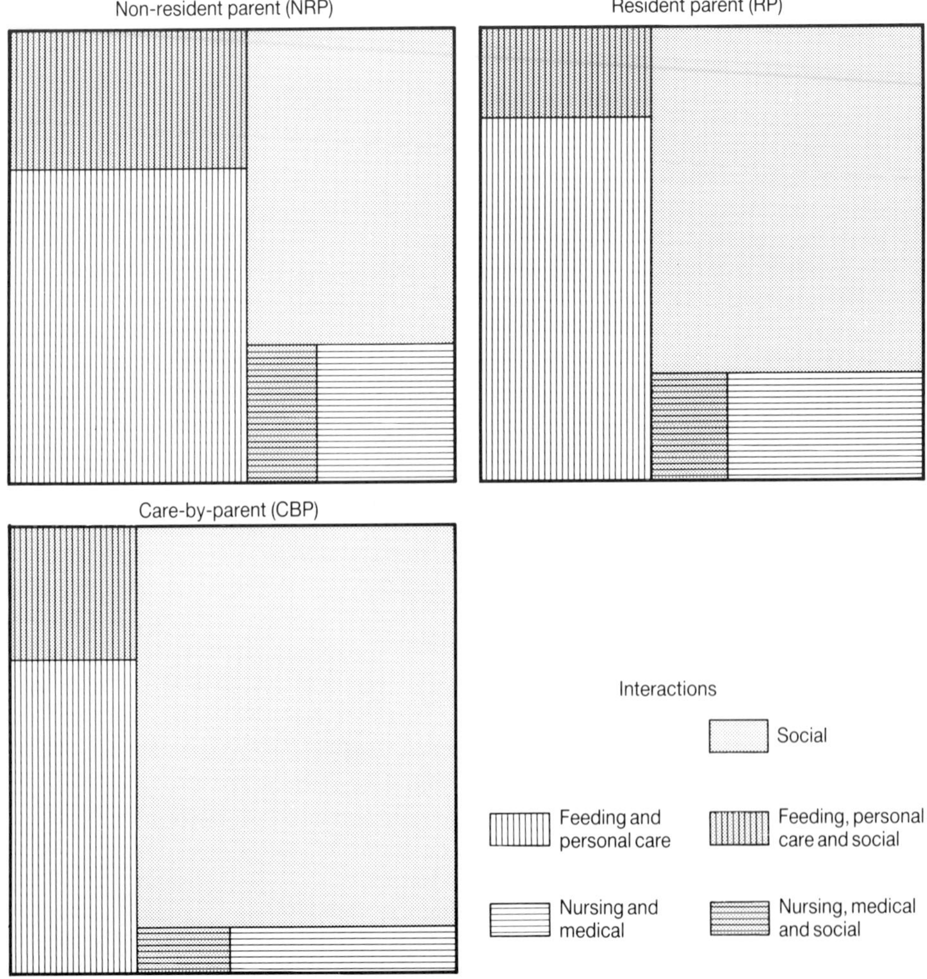

Figure 4.4 Nature of interactions: three care groups compared: percentage of total interactions

Table 4.4 Interactions with family and staff as a percentage

	NRP	RP	CBP
Interactions:			
With family	26.5	75.7	88.7
With staff	73.5	24.3	11.3
(n)	603	235	411

personal care, and less than one third are purely social (Figure 4.4). The figures for the CBP group are almost the reverse of this, and those for the RP group are intermediate. For all three groups, nursing and medical attention, which is, after all, the reason for being in hospital, was much the smallest category, although the most crucial elements (surgery and some investigations) would have taken place off the ward. Social interaction can be combined with the other kinds of activity, and the NRP children got more through this channel than did either of the other groups. Professionals may be better at combining two kinds of interaction than parents and may also realise how little social stimulation the children would get if staff did not take the opportunity when they had other duties to carry out. Interactions with the family are the most important for psychological well-being, and Table 4.4 gives the proportions of these.

The figures in Table 4.4 stress the success of care-by-parent in reducing the number of people handling a child, since 'staff' inevitably includes a large number of unfamiliar individuals, while family members rarely exceed half a dozen and will be well known to the child. Case allocation has improved the situation on the wards, but the needs of the hospital as workplace and educational establishment, as well as the changing case mix, may still mean that fairly large numbers of personnel are concerned in the care of one child. The records do not show precisely how many, because individuals cannot be identified without the observer's presence becoming intrusive. A nurse would be recorded as, for instance, staff nurse or student nurse, and not by name unless the observer happened to know it. However, in conjunction with the organisation of the working day, the records do give an idea of the numbers involved. One baby on one day received attention from at least three student nurses, two pupil nurses, a staff nurse, two sisters and a nursery nurse. An older child was seen with at least two staff nurses, an SEN, a sister, two student nurses and one pupil nurse.

For all groups the mother was the most important family contact, but for the NRP children both qualified nurses and learner nurses were more frequent contacts than any relative. CBP children saw less of nurses than did the RP group, but the main difference between the two groups with resident parents was that those in CBP saw more of other family members, especially their fathers, who sometimes took over from their mothers and visited more often. Siblings of CBP children also visited more often. The whole family may have felt more confident of having a rightful place in the ward, rather than being there on sufferance.

To sum up the lives of children in the Care-by-Parent Scheme, it is fair to say that they were mainly cared for by their mothers, with fathers assisting or sometimes taking over, and, where there were siblings, they saw them more frequently. The children were alone less and had more social interaction, having 'an attachment figure available and responsible which gives [them] a strong and pervasive feeling of security' (Bowlby 1988). They cried less than the other groups, particularly when they were alone.

THE ROLE OF PARENTS IN CARE-BY-PARENT

The reactions of parents (and nurses) to care-by-parent will be discussed in the following chapters, but the part they played and what nurses taught them to do must be considered, as must their attitudes and the effect upon the children. It was not possible within this study to evaluate the skill with which parents carried out nursing procedures. Sainsbury et al (1986) asked nurses to assess performance for a series of parents, some of whom also took part in the case studies. They 'considered that the parents performed the tasks satisfactorily in 30 of the 32 cases. In 15 instances they considered that the standards were, in fact, better'.

Monahan and Schkade (1985) have made a systematic study of children in a care-by-parent unit and in a conventional nursing milieu. All the children were learning to walk for the first time after surgery, and they had to cope with casts, braces and axillary crutches. They compared the mothers' performance with that of the nurses on four factors: children's weight loss (which is common), skin condition and urine collection, by catheter and by collection bag. Mothers performed as well as the nurses in all except the last category: both groups produced more contaminated specimens with the urine collection bag than with catheterisation, but mothers did somewhat less well than nurses with the bag.

The diary records of the present study include many accounts of mothers and fathers being shown how to do observations and chart them, or doing them on their own. They were also seen checking infusions and carrying out nasopharyngeal suction, and one mother was observed changing a tracheostomy inner tube. Some fathers took over from mothers at times – Emma's mother looked after her during the day, while her father stayed with her at night, when his wife went home to their other children. Peter's mother and father alternated on a 24-hour basis, and one grandmother also took part in care-by-parent. A few, mainly very young, fathers were too inexperienced at handling their own babies to manage on their own, so that CBP had to be suspended when the mothers went home. Sean's father was only 17, and was said, somewhat scornfully, to have had difficulty putting up a Z-bed. On the other hand, he could manage an apnoea alarm and learned what to do, including mouth-to-mouth resuscitation, if the alarm went off.

EXAMPLES FROM THE CASE STUDIES

There is more detail in some of the 21 case studies, although observers suspected that some self-conscious parents avoided doing things until they were on their own. However, Emma's mother was seen taking temperature, pulse and respiration, filling in the charts and using the nebuliser, singing to distract her from the noise it made. She was not pleased to find at 10 p.m. one night that an auxiliary nurse had already done the observations. This kind of confusion occasionally arose, particularly at night, but there was generally an easy relationship between parents and CBP nurses. Mothers might ask for a check on the way they had done something or hand over the responsibility when they took a break. Andrew's mother had taken some medication for a headache and gone to sleep early one night: Andrew was carefully removed from the cubicle when he awoke and fed elsewhere, in order not to disturb her. Staff were expected to see that mothers did not become overtired and that they sometimes got away from the ward.

Sarah (aged 16 months) was in hospital for investigation, including a jejunal biopsy, of a long-standing gut problem. Her mother had learned to do the usual observations and to record fluid intake and output, and she collected faecal specimens when required; she also had another child at home. In all three care groups, there were families with more than one child. Oddly, there were more in the two groups with resident parents (RP 5 out of 7 and CBP 7 out of 9) than in the NRP group (4 out of 10). Most of them had relatives or friends and neighbours who could help look after brothers and sisters. Unlike them, Sarah and her family had moved a good deal because of her husband's job and had only recently arrived in the area; her husband, a store manager, used to take the other daughter to work with him. The question of how families coped is considered in the next chapter.

Two children, Kenneth and Andrew, were the subjects of case studies at both periods of observation; accounts of their stays and the effect of care-by-parent have been assembled, using all the available data.

Case study 1

Kenneth is a representative of the older system of parent participation as well as of care-by-parent. He was a child with many congenital handicaps and, when the research team first saw him, was suffering from the effects of necrotising enterocolitis and had a ileostomy. He was brain damaged

Table 4.5 Kenneth: life in conventional nursing care

	% of time observed (n[1] = 2756)		
	Awake	Asleep	Total
Alone	3.2	10.3	13.5
With someone	63.1	23.4	86.5
Total	66.3	33.7	100.0

[1]n = 2756 10-second slots during 92 sets of 5-minute observations

with very little voluntary movement. The main consideration was to control fitting and frequent vomiting. His mother, who had an older child as well, stayed with Kenneth nearly all the time and already carried out many nursing procedures, necessary if he were to live at home. Having these skills at home was particularly important because, although they did not live very far away, it was an awkward journey by public transport, which could take 2 hours.

His mother had learned nasogastric feeding (including passing the tube), giving medication by the same route and nasopharyngeal suction, as well as stoma care and maintaining a special diet. Between the two observation periods the stoma was reversed and normal bowel function restored, although diarrhoea was often a problem. Kenneth's mother felt that this reversal had made a tremendous difference to their lives, since his problems were less conspicuous and journeys from home could be made without the difficulties of disposal or leakage associated with a stoma.

Kenneth's learning difficulties and lack of muscle tone meant that, unlike Andrew, there was very little difference in his pattern of behaviour at the two stages, as Tables 4.5 and 4.6 show. He cried rather more at the second stage – 8.8% of the time awake, but only 0.2% when he was alone. Although

Table 4.6 Kenneth: life in the Care-by-Parent Scheme

	% of time observed (n[1] = 3042)		
	Awake	Asleep	Total
Alone	2.8	8.9	11.7
With someone	62.3	26.0	88.3
Total	65.1	34.9	100.0

[1]n = 3042 10-second slots during 102 sets of 5-minute observations

Table 4.7 Kenneth: conventional care and care-by-parent compared: events as % of case study observation periods

	Conventional care (n[1] = 92)		Care-by-parent (n[1] = 102)	
Care by:	Parent	Professional[2]	Parent	Professional
Feeding, personal care	3.3	–	9.8	1.0
Reading/writing notes	–	2.2	11.8	2.0
Nursing:				
Professional only	n/a	6.5	n/a	3.9
Both: stoma care	9.8	1.1	n/a	n/a
other nursing	9.8	3.3	17.6	13.7
Discussion[3]/teaching	8.7		13.7	

[1]n = The number of sets of 5-minute observations
[2]'Professional' includes nurses, doctors and physiotherapists
[3]'Discussion' excludes what was described as chat or was purely social in character

his mother (and to a certain extent his father) had already learned many nursing procedures, there were some differences in the parents' involvement when they joined the Care-by-Parent Scheme. The main difference from the mother's point of view was that she now had responsibility for the care she was already competent to carry out and was expected, rather than allowed, to do it and enter it in the notes (Table 4.7). Kenneth needed both nasogastric and normal feeding – at which he was very slow; he also had to have nasopharyngeal suction, but did not need intravenous infusion or stoma care. New procedures, which his mother did in hospital for the first time, were taking his temperature, pulse and respiration, and the administration of oxygen.

Discussions with staff increased by more than half, but in the post-discharge interview, the mother said that she felt that she had less contact than before. This may have been because they were admitted to Central Ward, rather than the familiar North Ward, and to a cubicle at the far end of the corridor, past the playroom and the treatment room, so that neither staff nor visitors passed by. She also missed easy access to the parents' lounge, although she could still use it.

Kenneth's second admission lasted for 3 weeks, and at first he was too ill to be considered for care-by-parent. The observers had the impression that his mother was more depressed about the outlook for her son than she had been 6 months previously, when she was impatiently waiting for the stoma reversal. At that time she had been a great strength to several other young mothers, including Andrew's, who were coping with handicapped babies. Now, she and the mother in the adjoining cubicle, whose son also had severe fitting problems, were of great mutual support, sharing care and knowledge.

Case study 2

Andrew, the other child who was a case study patient at both periods of observation, was first seen at the age of 4 weeks, during activity sampling. Readmitted at around 6 weeks, his mother agreed to his becoming one of the case study children. At the second stage of observations, when he was about 8 months old, his mother joined the Care-by-Parent Scheme.

Stage I

Andrew had spent most of his 6 weeks in hospital, having had only a few days at a time at home. His mother always stayed with him, except for an occasional night at home; she was young and single, living with her own family at this time.

Andrew had developed flocculent hydrocephalus and the diagnosis was confirmed during the first case study period. The research records mention urine and stool collection, testing hearing and vision, measuring head circumference and keeping the mother informed. She said to an observer, 'They're still doing tests, I think they are hoping to reach a decision soon.' On the third day of the admission, the diagnosis was passed on; late in the afternoon, a doctor was recorded examining Andrew and talking to his mother, with contributions from a nurse. The observer also wrote that the mother 'was visibly upset towards the end of the five minutes. Nurse touched [her] consolingly' (28.10: 4.40 p.m.). Later she was described as 'still wandering up and down the corridor'. The case study period ceased shortly before Andrew had a shunt inserted, the first of many operations, and he went home a few days later, though not for very long.

Although she had spent so much time in hospital, Andrew's mother was never seen involved in his nursing care in any way, except for reading his notes on one occasion. She did observe and adapt to hospital practice in an appropriate manner: at first when Andrew's dummy fell on the floor, she sucked it herself (in the time-honoured fashion) before giving it back to him. Later, she washed it under the tap instead, and, before the end of the observations, she kept clean replacements in sterilising fluid.

Andrew was seldom left on his own, and when he was miserable or wanted attention he got an affectionate response. Table 4.8 gives the broad outline of his life in hospital. He was awake for a little less than half the time, and awake and alone for a very small proportion of that. The records show that he was crying for just over 10% of his waking time and less than half of that when he was alone. Crying alone occurred most often when his mother had been persuaded to take a break or go home for the night.

Table 4.8 Andrew: life in conventional nursing care

	% of time observed (n[1] = 4140)		
	Awake	Asleep	Total
Alone	6.5	37.1	43.5
With someone	40.0	16.5	56.5
Total	46.4	53.6	100.0

[1]n = 4140 slots during 138 sets of 5-minute observations

Andrew's mother appeared alarmed, almost repelled, by another boy with hydrocephalus, admitted a few days after Andrew's diagnosis had been confirmed. Simon was now 14 months old and his condition had proved difficult to control: his head was much enlarged and hampered his movements. In common with many mothers on the ward, Andrew's mother's chief support was Kenneth's mother.

Stage II

When the Care-by-Parent Scheme was being planned, Sister Eden immediately thought of Andrew's mother as someone who would be able to cope with it and benefit from it. She had experienced several more admissions and, sadly, it was virtually certain that there would be others before long. They were admitted about half way through the second observation period. Andrew's shunt had again blocked and the situation was complicated by a chest infection. This admission lasted for 5 weeks and he was the subject of a case study for two periods, of 7 and 5 days respectively.

As predicted, Andrew's mother liked the idea of CBP and quickly developed both competence and confidence. By the end of the observations, she had learned to do (and record) temperature, pulse and respiration – 'Easy, I've watched it being done so often' – to watch infusions and fill the burette, prepare and give nasogastric feeds and medication, as well as oral medication, and carry out nasopharyngeal suction. By the time of the post-discharge interview she had also learned to pass the nasogastric tube, although she confessed more than a year later that doing it still made her nervous. She accompanied Andrew to X-ray and other departments, including the operating theatre, and brought him back from the recovery room.

During this second set of observations there were changes in the pattern of the child's life, some due his increased age – that he was awake more, for example. The two periods of 7 days and 5 days have been treated as one, because the break was caused by anticipated surgery, which did not take

Table 4.9 Andrew: life in the Care-by-Parent Scheme

	% of time observed (n[1] = 6393)		
	Awake	Asleep	Total
Alone	9.5	27.7	37.2
With someone	45.6	17.2	62.8
Total	55.1	44.9	100.0

[1]n = 6393 10-second slots during 214 sets of 5-minute observations

place. Table 4.9 shows that the proportions of sleeping and waking were reversed. Andrew was alone less overall, but slightly more often when he was awake. However, a good many of the 'Alone, Awake' observations relate to occasions when his mother was hoping that he would go to sleep. Andrew cried a little more of his waking time, nearly 12%, but only 2% when he was alone:

5.05 p.m. Mother returned from dayroom with Andrew and placed him in cot. A little unsettled, but began to play with cot beads. Mother left briefly, (came back), checked that all was well, went out again. Andrew a little bit miserable, but settling down. (Diary 27.5)

There are noticeable differences in the mother's involvement in the two periods. In CBP she carried out over two-thirds of the nursing care, which was greater in total at this stage, partly because Andrew was on 2-hourly observations and, some of the time, on intravenous infusion. Table 4.10 gives some details.

The only occasion on which Andrew was seen being fed by a nurse was when his mother had gone home for the night. The time spent in discussion (a very small part of the observed talk was pure teaching) increased greatly, not only because it was now more necessary, but also because it was more valuable with an informed mother.

Andrew's mother was rarely out of earshot, even when he was alone, as she was probably in the parents' lounge or talking with other mothers elsewhere in the ward. Her friends in the ward now included Simon's mother, and she no longer found the look of him disturbing.

When she was persuaded to go out, her absence might still be quite brief. One day Staff Nurse said that she had gone out for the afternoon, but she was back by 2.45 p.m.; these trips usually ended in new clothes or toys for Andrew. Her plans were sometimes frustrated by non-cooperation from Andrew. One Saturday night, his mother had changed by 7.20 p.m. to go out for the evening. She was reluctant to leave before he went to sleep, so it was

Table 4.10 Andrew: conventional care and care-by-parent compared: events as % of case study observation periods

	Conventional care (n[1] = 138)		Care-by-parent (n[1] = 214)	
Care by:	Mother	Professional[2]	Mother	Professional[2]
Feeding, personal care	8.0	2.9	7.0	0.5
Reading/writing notes	0.7	5.8	7.0	4.7
Nursing:				
Professional only	n/a	7.2	n/a	5.1
Both	–	–	15.9	2.3
Discussion[3]/teaching	10.9		16.8	

[1]n = The number of sets of observations
[2]'Professional' includes nurses, doctors and physiotherapists
[3]'Discussion' excludes what was described as chat or was purely social in content

after 9 p.m. before she was persuaded to leave him with the nurses, and she was back by 10.30 p.m.

Her confidence extended beyond carrying out nursing procedures to querying doctors' decisions. A planned operation was postponed because of his chest condition, after she had spent the morning pushing a hungry baby in a theatre gown up and down the ward – the final decision did not reach her until after 1 p.m. It was then proposed to wait a month and do further tests before operating. She argued against the delay, being worried about increasing ventricular pressure, supporting her view by quoting the neurosurgeon and the state of the fontanelle. She heard a few days later, via Sister Eden, that the neurosurgeons would make a decision after the weekend. She regarded Sister Eden very much as an advocate and friend, while she herself became a great support to other mothers in the scheme in subsequent admissions and a great propagandist for it. Her role as support and informant was recognised within the Paediatric Unit, and the mothers of new babies with hydrocephalus were sent to her for information and reassurance.

LIFE IN THE 8-BEDDER

Case study children who were patients in Central rather than North Ward were in cubicles, so observation of the 8-bedder was incidental, but observers noted a strange situation developing there, because of one sad girl. Maria was admitted for periods of 3, 4 and 5 days. Aged 12, she had been brain-damaged by illness a few years before and now suffered from many cognitive defects, losing the ability to speak. She was very uncooperative and often aggressive, and her behaviour was sometimes bizarre. The other children (and their parents) found her frightening, while the staff viewed her arrival with trepidation, because she was unbiddable and unpredictable. On the weekend of activity sampling when occupancy was not very high, all the other children were moved, one by one, into the cubicles and Maria was left the only occupant, free to try all the beds in turn, as she liked to do.

A toddler, Brian, was admitted with a chest infection, while his mother was a patient in a surgical ward. The older girls in the ward spent a lot of time mothering him, but occasionally lost interest, so that he might find himself in a pram at the far end of the corridor.

The veterans Lucy and Paul were both patients again. Lucy had had quite a long period at home, but now had to have several stretches of intravenous infusion, which bitterly disappointed her. Her severely handicapped brother visited her several times and, although he could not walk, he could, and did, crawl effectively. Several mothers found the sight of a 14-year-old crawling along the corridor alarming, and hastily called their children away. Paul had had a bad winter and his mother was desperately hoping for some improvement in his condition.

Otherwise, there were similarities to stage 1 in the general pattern of behaviour, with pairs of inseparable small girls and groups of little boys inclined to rush about noisily.

A bigger boy, perhaps 10 years old, in the cubicle nearest C8, had panicked when he was due for surgery and resisted attempts to take him to theatre. The following day, after discussion including a psychiatrist and the boy's mother, the anaesthetist arrived on the ward. He explained what he was going to do and, after some commotion, induced unconsciousness in the cubicle, and the boy was wheeled off to theatre. Sister praised his mother; other nurses praised the anaesthetist, but in the 8-bedder the children played their radio, very loudly.

REFERENCES

Bowlby J (1988) *A Secure Base: Clinical Applications of Attachment Theory*. London: Tavistock/Routledge.

Cleary J (1979) Demands and responses: the effects of the style of work allocation on the distribution of nursing attention, in Hall DJ & Stacey M (eds.), *Beyond Separation*, pp. 109–127. London: Routledge & Kegan Paul.

Monahan GH & Schkade JK (1985) Comparing care by parent and traditional nursing units. *Pediatric Nursing*, **11**: 463–7.

Sainsbury CPQ, Gray OP, Cleary J, Davies MM & Rowlandson PH (1986) Care by parents of their children in hospital. *Archives of Disease in Childhood*, **61**: 612–16.

FURTHER READING

Casey A (1988) A partnership with child and family. *Senior Nurse*, **8**(4): 8–9.

Hall DJ (1987) Social and psychological care before and during hospitalisation. *Social Science and Medicine*, **25**: 721–32.

Jennings P (1988) Nursing and home aspects of the care of a child with tracheostomy. *Journal of Laryngology and Otology*, Supplement 17: 25–9.

Robertson J & Robertson J (1989) *Separation and the Very Young*. London: Free Association Books.

5

Parents' Experience of Participation and Care-by-Parent

It is clear that, during the observation period and follow-up, the Care-by-Parent Scheme was a success in objective terms: the nursing procedures were carried out adequately, or better, in nearly every case and the children cried less, had more social interaction and spent less time alone. These facts on their own would not ensure that the scheme was a significant contribution to the hospital care of children unless those most involved in carrying it out, the parents and staff, found satisfaction in their roles.

Although Jennings (1986) estimated that there were 13 CBP units in the USA and Canada, there is surprisingly little evidence about these aspects of the schemes. The published material (e.g. Fore & Holmes 1983, Oberlander 1980, Tonkin, 1979) mainly gives accounts of how the various units work, with general statements about attitudes and a few anecdotes about individuals. In the Lexington study (Lerner et al 1972), the great majority of parents, both those interviewed while they were in the hospital and those interviewed at home post-discharge, preferred the CBP unit because of its 'home-like atmosphere' and 'the way the parents and patients were treated'. Nearly all of the parents (46 out of 54) had to make arrangements for the care of other children, but interviews with a small group (13) of the partners who stayed at home reported only minimal problems due to CBP when compared to those caused by the illness or hospitalisation itself.

Caldwell and Lockhart (1981) report on parents' attitudes to taking part in care-by-parent at the University of Texas Medical Branch, Galveston. All admissions to the unit were planned, and it had no nursing personnel. Parents were asked to give their attitudes to their role in caring for their children. Over 80% gave the highest possible positive rating to statements about whether they felt 'comfortable', 'confident' and 'satisfied with the care' and that they did not 'feel confined'. There was more variation in answers to changes in their feelings during their stay, suggesting that some parents were well used to their nursing role and so experienced no change. The most frequent responses to questions about what they had liked most and least about their stay were 'being able to stay with [their] child' (142; 91.6%) and 'became bored' (20; 12.9%). The lower cost of CBP was mentioned by nearly two-thirds of parents.

The financial advantages of CBP are mentioned in nearly all the American articles and are dealt with comprehensively by Evans and Robinson (1983) for the unit in Vancouver. During the Cardiff research period, it was not possible to estimate how the introduction of the Care-by-Parent Scheme affected the budget of the Paediatric Unit within the wards taking part. Current accounting methods would probably shed more light on the subject.

Cost was not a factor in the scheme described by Monahan and Schkade (1985, see also p.58). Two CBP groups (5 days intensive gait training or regular therapy to an agreed standard) and two similar control groups, conventionally nursed, were studied. All the families had had considerable experience of hospitalisation. Those in both the intensive groups, particularly the CBP mothers, showed increasing anxiety, unlike the regular groups. However, nearly all the CBP mothers reported great satisfaction with the time they could spend with their children. In a smaller study (Monahan & Schkade 1986, in correspondence with the author), 24 CBP mothers reported that they felt comfortable caring for their children, and nearly all were satisfied with the nursing supervision. All but one would recommend CBP to other parents:

> I feel that this opportunity to be in on this program has hastened my son's recovery 100%.

> I think this unit was better than any hospital stay we have ever had. I would most definitely recommend this to any parent I know. I would make no change. Thanks a million.

The only negative comments concerned physical conditions or restrictions on activity, apart from a plaintive 'make mothers compatible'.

In the present study, questionnaires were administered to parents of case study children in the post-discharge interviews, and observers recorded informal conversations with them. The confidentiality of their responses was stressed; neither the author nor the other interviewer (Greta Thomas) were employed by the hospital, and all the data were to be stored and analysed in another town.

THE PARENTS AT THE FIRST OBSERVATION PERIOD

The children who were case studies in the first stage of observation were chosen because they had conditions which would have been appropriate for CBP, rather than because their parents were keen on the idea. The records and post-discharge interviews with 17 of them showed that nine had parents (mother, father or sharing) who were resident throughout and another

(Martin's) was present for 1 week of a 3-week admission; the five oldest children were admitted alone. Martin was 6½ months, and his mother thought his behaviour after an earlier admission meant that visiting would be sufficient after he had settled in. She was disappointed to find that this time he was upset when he came home again. Stacey P (see Chapter 2) was one of the youngest children alone. Her single mother would have liked to have spent more time visiting and, ideally, to have stayed, but found it impossible because of the cost, the distance and having to bring her 2-year-old with her – who had to be amused and kept out of trouble.

Charles, aged 11 months, was in hospital for a week, and his mother was one of the very few who really did not want to visit more, or stay or be involved in his care in hospital. His condition was not life-threatening but required meticulous attention to personal care and diet. Asked whether she had carried out any of the nursing care, she said, 'I was gone by then', and at various times, 'I can't stand hospitals' and child care 'gets on my nerves'. She did not expect to spend all the time with him when she did visit or go to him if he cried. It was noticeable that her son slept much less than most of the children on North Ward, being described as wary or watchful rather than as displaying distress. He was a responsive, sociable child, who attracted a lot of casual attention from passers-by, and he was recorded spending more time with nurses than with his mother. Predictably, his behaviour when he went home was very disturbed; his mother said 'Yes – yes – yes – all of that' as the interviewer went through the list of adverse reactions, and she volunteered that he was crying all the time. He also bit her hand very hard as she went to do up a button on his coat during the interview.

The 4- and 5-year-old children in the non-resident group were in Central Ward, and some of them had been present during the activity sampling as well (see Chapter 3). Paul's mother was another who hated hospitals, but she visited for 8 or 9 hours a day, 'as much as I can cope with', while Lucy's mother very much regretted that the needs of her handicapped son meant that she had never been able to stay; distance and transport were also a difficulty for her. The other 5½-year-old had diabetes, and his mother, who had stayed with him when he was younger, now wanted him to learn to cope independently with his condition and its consequences. They lived further away than most, and she said, 'A couple of years ago, when my husband wasn't working, I'd go all day without food to afford the fare.'

The parents of the remaining two, who were 7 and 9 years old, thought it unnecessary to stay with children of that age: Louise's mother said, 'She's better on her own', a view that the observers would have disputed.

Among the parents of these case study children, over half were resident for all or part of the time with the child in hospital, and another two would have liked to be resident. In 1978 (Royal Commission on the NHS 1978) little more than a quarter of the sample stayed or would have liked to. Whether this difference was due to a change in the climate of opinion or to local variations in parents' attitudes and hospital policy is a matter of conjecture.

The case study parents were asked whether they could carry out any of the care that their own child had received and whether they would be prepared to take the responsibility for what they did. Those whose children had chronic conditions had already learned to do many things, and most of them were prepared to do more and take responsibility for them in hospital, as they already did at home. Andrew (see Chapter 4) was about 8 weeks old at the time, and his mother was prepared to take on anything she had seen done for him – and did, by the time he was 6 months older. Charles' mother, predictably, did not want the responsibility. Nearly all of the others were prepared to do more, although few of them were aware of the kind of procedures some mothers (like Kenneth's, see Chapter 4) were already carrying out at home. One was afraid of the responsibility, and a few felt that they would be slow in gaining the necessary confidence. Paul's mother saw his time in hospital as some slight respite from the constant stress of the regime that cystic fibrosis demands, although while she was with him she attended to the drip, administered the nebuliser and did some physiotherapy, as well as keeping him amused.

The 'best thing' recorded about the admission was either being able to stay or visit as often and as long as they liked, coupled with the attitude of the nurses, or some aspect of recovery, or simply 'going home'. The 'worst thing' produced two kinds of response: either worry about the illness or the distress that treatment caused, or some aspect of hospitalisation, rather than the illness, and lead on to other aspects of the stay. Boredom was mentioned by several parents – 'the days go so slowly', said Andrew's mother – as was the meals being so far away. Some found the restrictions on space their biggest problem, particularly when children were barrier nursed. Those who were resident gave 'missing other children at home' as the worst thing, and those who were not resident, 'missing the one in hospital'; the complication of reconciling the needs of the child in hospital with those of the family at home was also mentioned, particularly when transport was a problem.

Practically all these mothers believed that their children had a great need for them when they were in hospital. Those who did not stay or visit very much were more often constrained by family and economic circumstances rather than making a free choice.

Although one mother clung to the old idea that children were spoiled in hospital, the largest group of these parents considered that their children were upset by being in hospital, although older children might be said just to 'put up with it'. Two of the older children who had had frequent admissions were thought to 'quite enjoy it', others to 'settle down quickly', another phrase from the past. Attempts to interview some of the older children were not very productive: the Consumers' Association (1980) reported similar difficulties but gives the results of some interviews with young patients by a child psychologist.

CARE-BY-PARENT

The parents of the CBP children all expected to stay with their children in hospital, although one was unable to make arrangements for her other child for the first night. Presumably, they were all part of the majority who considered it necessary to stay with a young child in hospital and to that extent were self-selected. The post-discharge questionnaire (see the Appendix) was administered either at the hospital, when the child had a follow-up appointment, or at home 2 to 4 weeks after discharge. Three families out of the 24 could not be contacted. The questionnaire covered aspects of the child's health and reactions to hospital as well as the parents' attitudes and experience of parental involvement and CBP.

General attitude to CBP

Asked whether they thought that CBP was a good idea and whether they would want to be in the scheme again, 19 of the 21 respondents said 'yes' to both questions. The one grandmother who took part was the primary care-giver for a child with severe congenital handicaps, thought it was a good idea but felt that the responsibility was perhaps too great.

The one dissenting mother (Matthew's) had very ambivalent views – on the one hand that it was a good idea and that she wanted to do as much as possible for the child herself, but on the other that the nurses ought to be doing it as it was their job. She was very young and single, very much on the defensive: 'Because I am young, they think I am not a proper mother'. Her manner was somewhat aggressive and she complained loudly about what she regarded as shortcomings on the part of nurses. She was little older than, say, some of the fibrocystic patients seen in the unit, but some staff did not seem disposed to make allowances for her youth and inexperience; the relations between them went from bad to worse, staff finding her unreasonable and unappreciative, she regarding them as uncaring and disapproving. It was an unhappy situation and difficult to rectify within the day-to-day running of the ward.

Two of the mothers were qualified nurses who would have been carrying out most of the care anyway. Their confidence was not increased by participation in CBP, but 13 of the other parents said theirs was. Two mothers commented that they had now dealt with an illness in another of their children easily, 'when before I would have panicked' as one of them put it (they both used the word 'panic'). Those who described their confidence as being the same either already did a great deal at home and found no great change or, during a fairly brief admission, had not taken on anything which seemed to them out of the ordinary. Parents' views about the nature and scope of CBP was always coloured by what they themselves had done, not realising the complexity and perilous nature of the procedures carried out by some mothers, and they would probably have been appalled at the prospect. Geraint's mother had learned to do a tremendous amount for her child, now 12, including managing a Hickman's catheter. She commented 'If someone had said to you at the beginning, "You're going to be doing this and this and this", I'd have said, "Don't be so ridiculous, I could never do it" – the furthest thing from my mind was anything to do with nursing!' Her understanding and skill in coping with her son's condition and needs were acknowledged by both medical and nursing staff. She had begun learning long before CBP started. The only parent who reported no improvement in confidence, which was already not high, was the husband of one of the nurse/mothers, who shared the care with his wife and found that staff tended to assume that he needed very little instruction.

Responsibility for care

Parents were asked whether they found CBP too much of a tie or too great a responsibility, since once in the scheme, their presence and participation in care was essential rather than casual. Only a few considered that it was sometimes too much of a tie or that some things could be too much responsibility, but they viewed this as being for others rather than themselves or if their own child had been more seriously ill. No-one felt that what he or she had actually taken on was too much. The overall impression was that the responsibility for the child was the parent's, no matter who was carrying out the care, and CBP gave them the opportunity to discharge their obligations. Whether the stress of added responsibility for care might be insupportable for some individuals, even though they found satisfaction in being actively involved, is a question which needs further investigation. Meantime, it is important that nurses encourage parents to take care of themselves as well as their children.

Parents' breaks

Parents were asked how they organised breaks for themselves, but it must be acknowledged that the question was interpreted in two ways. Those whose children were in hospital for no more than 2 or 3 days thought basically in terms of meal breaks and worried about the distance to the dining room, while those involved in admissions that went on for weeks rather than days had to think of breaks to attend to family and household matters as well as their own needs for change and relief, not just food. Short-stay parents took breaks when the child was asleep (13 parents) and/or another relative was there (9 parents). Some had meals brought in so that they would not have to leave the child. Two mothers said that they just 'didn't feel like eating' and rarely went further than the parents' room or the telephone – 'I don't want her to wake up while I am away and be frightened.' Those who needed to leave the hospital for a few hours or overnight usually did so when the father was sharing care or a grandmother could stand in for an afternoon. Otherwise, they checked carefully with Sister (who might well be urging the outing) that a nurse would take over in their absence. This was particularly important for the baby with the tracheostomy, whose mother never left the ward without telling the staff. She said, of other parents rather than herself, that where children were particularly demanding during the day, night staff should do more and let the parents rest. In informal conversation, she confessed that in some ways she preferred another local hospital, where nurses took over the care and she got some relief from the treadmill of hourly suctioning.

One father, who shared care, said that he 'tended to go without [breaks], took sandwiches because [I] couldn't get her to sleep.'

On the whole, staff encouraged those who stayed more than a few days to get out of the ward; one mother said that 'nurses came in and asked if [I] wanted to pop out'. Sometimes nurses would take children for a ride around the unit in their pushchairs or up to the concourse to give the parents an opportunity for a meal or TV programme undisturbed.

Facilities for parents

Parents were asked for their opinions of the facilities for parents and specifically about meals and sleeping arrangements. Most of the comments were about meals and the distance to the dining rooms, which were, undoubtedly, about as far away as they could be. Twelve respondents regarded the distance as a great disadvantage, taking them away from their children for too long, although another said that it was 'good in one respect, gives you a walk and a break'. Two people had their main meals brought in rather than be away that much. Opinions of the food itself, which was, at that time, of a rather institutional kind, ranged from 'nice' and 'OK', through 'not too bad, considering the price' and 'not very good' to 'like school dinners' (from a teacher), 'disgusting' and 'atrocious' from the two nurse/mothers.

Judgements about the sleeping facilities were much more uniformly favourable, although a folding bed, for one parent only, in a small cubicle is not the most comfortable arrangement. Nineteen of the 21 respondents gave moderate or enthusiastic replies from 'all right' to 'marvellous', mainly because they were beside their children: 'You can't ask for more than being right there in the cubicle.' The advantages of being in the same room were stressed particularly by those who had experience of other hospitals, where parents' accommodation was seldom available on the ward. Noise, a common complaint in hospitals, was mentioned only once.

They seldom referred to the parents' room, bathroom and kitchen on North Ward, perhaps taking these amenities for granted. The facilities were not luxurious but there were armchairs and a TV set, and the opportunity to take a shower or make cups of tea whenever they wanted. Kenneth's mother missed easy access to them and felt somewhat isolated when he was admitted to Central Ward.

CARE FOR OTHER CHILDREN

Arranging care for children other than the patient is an anxiety shared by many resident parents. Five of the nine parents resident during the first observation period had one or more other children. In three families, they were looked after by grandmothers, and in another the unemployed father was the resident parent. A burly, unkempt looking man, he was notably gentle and playful with his small daughter. For the last, care was provided by someone outside the family. Six of the non-resident parents had other children and three gave this as a reason for not staying.

Among the CBP case study group, 11 of the 21 families had more than one child. One grandmother was the resident carer and two others looked after the other children, while six families shared care between mother and father. One father managed with the help of friends, and one took the child to work with him. Others took time off work, either as holiday or unpaid leave, and one was on strike. Fathers were more often involved in their children's care, for both those at home and those in hospital, among the CBP group. These parents were clear in their own minds that the needs of the sick child in hospital were greater than those of the healthy ones at home, although one mother, resident for many weeks, described herself as 'torn between them'.

COSTS TO FAMILIES

All the families found that having a child in hospital caused considerable extra expense, even though the health care was free. Resident or non-resident, there were travel costs, petrol or bus and taxi fares; sharing care or ferrying other children to grandmothers might mean several trips in a day. Meals in hospital also cost more than meals at home.

The child in hospital often needed new night or day clothes and, as a rule, was given daily presents of toys and sweets to help pass the time. Care for siblings might involve expense as well, and they usually got consolation presents.

Direct financial loss occurred when fathers and mothers took unpaid time off work. These losses ranged from £20–£250, the highest figure being for a supply teacher who turned down several jobs during CBP. Some of this loss would have occurred with a child ill at home, although fathers were less likely to have lost wages in such a case. The other expenses were estimated at between £8 and £40. A child whose chronic condition entails many hospital admissions can be a constant drain on the family resources, particularly if they live at a distance (Burton 1975).

COMMUNICATION AND INFORMATION

Problems of communication between staff and patients or their relatives and the difficulty of getting information have been the subject of discussion (and complaint) for many years and keep on recurring (Jones et al 1987). Parents in this study were asked about various aspects of obtaining information at both stages of the observations. Broadly, the questions covered three areas, two of them clinical (information about what was going to happen to the child, and the results of tests and their implications) and one practical (where to find what they and their child needed).

Most first stage parents felt that they had been given sufficient information about the need for admission, either by their own family doctor or at the hospital. The parents of 'veterans' were usually good judges of their children's state of health and brought them straight to the hospital if they were worried. The treatments and tests were familiar to these families and well explained to most of the rest. Where test results were involved, nine respondents said they got them quickly and five said they did not – 'Had to chase them.' Information about the implications for the child's future was satisfactory for just over half. The others were unhappy because the results of tests were inconclusive or they found the explanations unconvincing.

Some children had had three or more previous admissions and their parents knew where things were and what to do. Those whose children were admitted for the first time to this unit mainly said that they had to find these things out for themselves from staff or other mothers. Only three had been told what they needed to know without having to ask. One mother complained of getting inconsistent messages about what she was allowed to do and where she was allowed to go.

At the second follow-up stage, the questions about clinical and practical information were repeated, alongside questions specifically about the Care-by-Parent Scheme:

- whether it was well explained beforehand;
- whether the booklet was adequate;
- whether it was easy to find the CBP nurse;
- whether there was ever confusion about who was responsible for particular procedures;
- whether the teaching was well done or too much was expected too quickly.

About clinical matters, half felt that they had been given the information quickly and fully or that there was nothing new to say. The others were dissatisfied, as in the first stage, because inevitably some test results were inconclusive – 'they couldn't pinpoint the cause of Michelle's attack' (the first, of asthma) – or they felt that they only got answers by persistent questioning: Andrew's mother said, 'You had to take the initiative, the surgeons didn't volunteer information.' There were also complaints about slow results and 'doctors' language'. On the other hand, one experienced mother said, 'Getting information is good, now that the Care-by-Parent is going on.'

Satisfaction about practical matters was higher in CBP: nearly two-thirds were told, or already knew, what they needed to know, or found it in the CBP booklet.

Asked whether they thought that the Care-by-Parent Scheme had been well explained to them in the first instance, three quarters said 'yes', three parents said 'no' and two had some reservations. Michelle's mother said that when she asked what was going to happen to her child, she was told that they would 'try a few things'. It all seemed vague. She was surprised, looking back, that they asked her to take over (i.e. join CBP) when she didn't know what to expect.

The parents' booklet was given to parents at the time they were offered the option, to help them make their decision. This has gone through several revisions, and the version rewritten in the light of the research findings appears in the Appendix. The one distributed during the observation period was considered adequate by 14 respondents, 'lots of information in the booklet' (although one disliked the tone – 'too many orders') and poor by four – 'You need more than the booklet.' Inexplicably, three were never given it. One mother found it a life-saver, because she had been told quite inaccurately that there was nowhere for parents to get meals and she had been trying to exist on snacks and crisps from the WRVS.

FINDING THE CBP NURSE

The care-by-parent nurse on each shift was expected to be the teacher and provider of support and information to the parents, the linchpin of the scheme. He or she wore a badge like the one identifying the child's cubicle and needed to be easily accessible. When parents were asked whether they experienced problems finding the right nurse, the responses were very mixed, as shown in Table 5.1 (p.78). In some ways the third and fourth responses were the most worrying and suggested that the role of the CBP nurse was not being made clear or that there was too much variation in the way it was carried out. A mother who found no problems reported that they 'introduced themselves, they are always in and out'. One who did have difficulties said, 'If only the parent-care nurse could have kept popping in and out, saying "If you have any problems, I'm here," and introduced herself for the day.' Time and staff changes had something to do with this: most of the parents giving

Table 5.1 Were there problems finding the CBP nurse?

No problems	9
Yes – problems	4
Did not know there was one	4
Just asked any nurse	3
No need (mother a nurse)	1
Total	21

negative or inappropriate responses joined the scheme near the end of the observations. When what might be called the founder members were on leave or had moved on, some elements of the scheme, which was largely undocumented, began to lose their clarity and might be disregarded. Some competent parents still lacked confidence and needed more support.

TEACHING AND RELATIONSHIPS WITH NURSES

Parents were asked specifically about being taught to take temperature, pulse and respiration (TPR), because, at that time, these were the first things that parents were taught. Temperatures were taken rectally. The questionnaire asked whether it was done well (12 respondents said 'yes') or whether too much was expected too quickly. The main complaint from those who had already learned a great deal was, again, insufficient support. Kenneth's mother, who was already doing things as complex as nasopharyngeal suction, said she would have felt more confident if the nurses 'could have come in and helped the first few times', which was, of course, what they did with those they regarded as novices. Simon's mother felt that too much was expected too quickly; what she already knew had been learnt over many months. The mother who looked after a tracheostomy at home still wanted reassurance but said, 'The nurses – I hardly saw them.' Another less experienced mother said, 'That's why I had to keep calling the nurse in.' She, like the great majority, agreed that the nurse(s) who taught her were sympathetic and patient. Predictably, Matthew's mother did not, and another very young mother distinguished between the CBP nurses, who were helpful, and the others, who were not.

CONFUSION IN THE SCHEME

One of the problems which arose from the constantly shifting responsibility for CBP, and the lack of any prominent clue, was confusion about how much an individual parent had taken on. Seven parents reported that on one or more occasions, they found that a nurse had done something (usually giving medication or doing the TPR observations) without checking whether the parent was going to do them. They objected both because they felt that their contribution was being underrated and their precarious confidence undermined, and, more practically, that they were going to do the procedure at a time which fitted in with the child's own routine. On one occasion, an axillary temperature had been taken instead of a rectal one, so that a misleading value had been recorded. Most of these incidents occurred at night, with staff who were perhaps less well informed (at that time they did not rotate day staff) and possibly even hostile to the idea. Again, Matthew's mother was one of those involved and had something of an altercation over it.

HOW PARENTS SAW THEIR FUTURE INVOLVEMENT

At the follow-up interviews at both stages, parents were asked whether they thought that they could learn to do more in the way of nursing procedures for their children in hospital. They answered in the light of the care their own child had received.

Those who had been in CBP were more optimistic about their own abilities. The two nurse/mothers were able and willing to do anything they could envisage, although another nurse/mother, seen during the activity sampling, confessed that she found it difficult to do anything unpleasant to her own child. Two lay mothers felt that they wanted to do as much as possible and could learn anything on the list in the questionnaire (see the Appendix) and were willing to take the responsibility for it. Six more thought that they could learn some things but not all (one excepted giving injections, 'too squeamish', another managing intravenous infusions) or would prefer that nurses carried on with the more complex procedures. Michelle's mother said, 'No, I'm not cut out for it, it upsets me. If I had to, in an emergency, yes, but I'd rather the nurses did it.' She had 'not felt like eating' and had lost half a stone while her daughter was in hospital. The father had shared in the care as well as looking after the older brother. Both parents were contemplating the implications of the diagnosis of asthma, thinking in terms of coping better 'next time'. Another mother, whose daughter had had open heart surgery in another hospital by the time of the interview, felt quite overwhelmed by the technicalities. The only person who said that there would be too much responsibility for parents in general, rather than for herself, was the mother who was already doing tracheostomy care at home.

It is difficult to compare these opinions with those of the novice case study parents at the first stage of observation, because most of them found it difficult to imagine a situation in which they took over from the nurses in any sense. Four of the mothers with children under 4 years old, including Andrew's mother, felt that they could learn to do what they had seen being done and would be prepared to take the responsibility. Six others had more misgivings. Four of the older children had chronic conditions – asthma, diabetes or cystic fibrosis – and their parents were already expert in their home care. However, they were divided in their opinions, two of them thinking that it was logical and desirable to carry on with the child's care in hospital, and two that an in-patient admission was their only opportunity for respite, which is sad if true.

The parents who had been in the Care-by-Parent Scheme, despite some reservations about particular procedures, were almost unanimous that they would want to do it again if the same or another child was in hospital.

A STUDY OF PARENTS' ATTITUDES

In 1985–6, a study of parents' attitudes to their children's hospitalisation was carried out by Lee (1986), a postgraduate psychology student. In this she compared CBP parents, other resident parents (NCBP) and visiting parents (VP). The decision to be a visiting, rather than a resident, parent did not appear to be governed by objective considerations, such as other children or jobs. Neither these nor the seriousness of the illness (assessed by the paediatricians) were the determining factors. The choice was based on the family's beliefs about the needs of sick children. The consensus of the three groups was that children of 4 to 5 years could be independent in normal circumstances, but the visiting parents were less well informed than the others about the possible effects of hospitalisation on children. If their (VP) children were under 1 year old, they were likely to believe that they were too young to miss their parents.

Lee also used a standard research instrument, the General Health Questionnaire (Goldberg 1978), which is often used for comparing levels of stress between groups. Visiting parents showed significantly more stress than either of the other groups and the CBP group less than the NCBP.

Most children in the NCBP group were being admitted for the first time and hardly any of the parents had heard of care-by-parent, but all of them (26 NCBP respondents) said, after reading a short description of the scheme, that they would have liked to be in it. One said that a nursing procedure 'would not be something nasty if I did it, rather than someone else – he trusts me'. It is possible that the scheme was simply being operated erratically at that time, but it may be that having previously been a resident parent was being used as a criterion for joining CBP. Either having been a 'successful' resident parent in the past was considered as evidence of suitability or CBP was being offered principally to children who were likely to have repeated admissions.

The CBP parents all felt that they were contributing to the child's recovery and that the child was happier in the scheme. They also stressed the practical value of learning nursing skills which would be used at home. The results support the findings of the main study about parents' attitudes towards CBP, but they also indicate that less than 2 years after its inception, it was being implemented less widely and, perhaps, inconsistently.

PARENTS SUM UP

Some time after the end of the observation periods, a visiting lecturer in paediatric nursing asked the mother of a baby with Down's syndrome what she felt about CBP. She replied that she felt useful and not in the way, that she was able to do things at the right moment, and that she had felt anxious at first but was now more confident, although she still found the pulse difficult and always got the nurse to check it.

Another official visitor talked to a mother who had learned total parenteral feeding. She described how her skills had been built up slowly from the simple things at first – she could not have taken them on at the beginning. She had spent some time in another hospital and there, she said, 'I did not feel that he was my baby', and she was convinced that it was not good for children 'to have strangers doing things to them'. It was also very boring staying in hospital, if she had nothing to do and the baby was too ill to be responsive.

Writing to the author (copies of the case studies in Chapter 4 were sent to Andrew and Kenneth's parents, in case they wished to comment or objected to publication) in 1990, Andrew's mother said:

> Being part of the CBP scheme has played a vital role in helping me to cope with Andrew's illness. I have learnt to know when he needs to go to hospital, or if he isn't too bad (e.g. his pulse, temperature and respirations are OK), to keep him at home. Being on the CBP Scheme, I took part in helping Andrew and knowing I was helping him and not feeling useless made me feel better . . . I know that Andrew feels better if I or his dad do things for him, rather than a nurse. Although in the past 6 years we have found that all the nurses . . . have been very helpful.

REFERENCES

Burton L (1975) *The Family Life of Sick Children*. London: Routledge & Kegan Paul.

Caldwell BS & Lockhart LH (1981) A care-by-parent unit: its planning, implementation and patient satisfaction. *Children's Health Care*, **10**(1): 4–7.

Consumers' Association (1980) *Children in Hospital: a Which? Campaign Report*. London: Consumers' Association.

Evans RG & Robinson GC (1983) An economic study of cost savings on a care-by-parent ward. *Medical Care*, **21**: 768-82.

Fore CV & Holmes SS (1983) A care-by-parent unit revisited. *American Journal of Maternal/Child Nursing*, **8**: 408-10.

Goldberg D (1978) *Manual of the General Health Questionnaire*. Windsor: National Foundation for Educational Research.

Jennings K (1986) Helping them face tomorrow. *Nursing Times*, **82**(4): 33–5.

Jones L, Lenehan L & Maclean U (1987) *Consumer Feedback for the NHS*. London: King Edward's Hospital Fund for London.

Lee MS (1986) *Parents' Perception of and Response to the Hospitalization of their Children*. MSc Dissertation, University of Wales, Institute of Science and Technology.

Lerner MJ, Haley JV, Hall DS & McVarish D (1972) Hospital care-by-parent: an evaluative look. *Medical Care*, **X**: 430–6.

Monahan GH & Schkade JK (1985) Comparing care by parent and traditional nursing units. *Paediatric Nursing*, **11**: 463–8.

Oberlander R (1980) Parent care units bring home to hospital. *Hospitals*, **54**(21): 81–5.

Royal Commission on the National Health Service (1978) *Patients' Attitudes to the Hospital Service*. Research Paper no.5. London: OPCS.

Tonkin P (1979) Parent care for the low risk and terminally-ill child. *Dimensions in Health Service*, **56**: 42–3.

FURTHER READING

Cartwright A (1964) *Human Relations and Hospital Care*. London: Routledge & Kegan Paul.

Thornes R (1985) Parent participation. *Nursing Mirror*, **160**(13): 20, 22.

Thornes R (1987) Parental access and family facilities in children's wards in England. *British Medical Journal*, **287**: 190–2.

6

Nurses' Attitudes to the Care-by-Parent Scheme

Without the commitment of the nursing staff to the idea, and their wholehearted cooperation in running it, the Care-by-Parent Scheme would have had no hope of success, even in the short term. The Steering Committee were greatly disappointed that there was never sufficient funding to explore fully the impact of care-by-parent on the lives and work of the nurses. In the 1960s hospitals were slow to adopt unrestricted visiting because the effects on the ward nurse had been ignored. Ideally, this aspect would have been studied, alongside the observations of the children and their parents, in order to find out what they felt about their changing role. Was teaching and counselling as satisfying as hands-on care? How far did they think that parents were reliable and competent to take over care? Did sharing hard-won professional knowledge with lay people go against the grain? Did the new system increase or decrease the workload or simply shift it about? Did it require a different skill mix among staff? Was it practicable to offer CBP on a general ward or would it have been better to be more selective about the patients and restrict it to a separate unit? How were patients and parents selected in practice? These questions are still in need of detailed answers.

In order to get some idea of nurses' attitudes to increasing parental involvement before the scheme started, a self-completion questionnaire was devised (see the Appendix). Diary records of informal conversations and comments about the scheme were also kept. The following year a second student dissertation examined nurses' attitudes, and its findings are reported below (p. 91).

THE NURSES' QUESTIONNAIRE

The questionnaire covered the staff's ideas about children's reactions to being in hospital and need for the presence of their parents (or other relatives) at various ages, as well as the practicability of handing over nursing tasks to parents. There were 36 respondents, ranging in age from under 21 to over 50, with a great variety in the qualifications they held or were studying for (degree, DN, RSCN, SCM, RGN, SEN, NNEB), there being none in the case of two long-serving nursing auxiliaries. More than half of them had also worked outside nursing. Members of the permanent staff had worked in the unit for periods ranging from a few months to its entire existence. This tremendous variation among a relatively small, self-selected group means that a simple numerical analysis could be misleading, so the results are given in general terms. On the whole, those who had worked for longest in the unit, and those who were most highly qualified, had the greatest confidence in the abilities of parents. The nurses did agree (except for three of the learners) on one thing: they regarded paediatrics as one of the most interesting areas within nursing. The other specialties most frequently picked were obstetrics and special care baby work.

Everyone believed that 'children react differently to being in hospital at different ages', but the answers to more detailed questions suggested that they did not regard developmental stage to be as important as personality in their expectations of an individual child. All but the oldest SEN thought that children aged 1 to 4 years (inclusive) would be upset by admission to hospital, but ideas about younger and older children varied a great deal, and some did not reject the notion of 'settling down'.

There was a fair consensus about what the ideal was – that all the under-5s should have a relative to stay in hospital with them, and that mothers and fathers were the most appropriate people to stay. Older children were thought not to need resident parents, but there was a split in opinion about whether they should be visited 'all day' or 'for a few hours only'. Teenagers were almost universally held to need 'only a few hours each day', although one nursing auxiliary appeared to think it would be better if they had no visitors at all.

Asked whether the presence of parents on the ward affected their work, the great majority of the respondents (28 out of 36) said 'yes', and some who said 'no' made comments like 'There is not enough space to work comfortably together.' Many acknowledged the need to see the family as a whole and involve parents in the child's treatment, but others felt self-conscious or even threatened:

> Often the nurse is unable to be completely natural with the child when she is being watched by parents. However, the child is obviously much happier when parents are present. (Student nurse)

> They constantly watch and question what you do, but on the whole the advantages outweigh the disadvantages. (Recently qualified staff nurse)

> Not the permanent staff. Learners, however, are unused to it as a general rule, but most adjust well and quickly. (Sister)

Some felt that involving parents freed the nurses to spend more time with the other children:

> Gives the nurse more time to come and play with children without parents in the ward, by taking over many of the basic nursing tasks – feeding, hygiene, reassurance. (Student nurse)

However, one thought that there could be dangers in this:

> The nurse may not always react to the parents' presence in the ward in the best way That is she may not attend to the child as she sees the parents as carrying out his requirements, not bothering to find out if the parents are coping with this and are giving the correct care. (Undergraduate nurse)

This parallels the opinions of the parents who wanted more support with the new responsibilities they were undertaking.

Everyone agrees that child (and adult) patients have psychological and social needs and that it is part of the job of the nurses and other specialist staff to try to meet them, particularly in the absence of relatives. It is also clear that meeting these needs does not, and could not, take precedence over clinical matters, although the latter may provide an opportunity for psychological care, since play and comforting can often be combined with nursing and personal care. It is something that requires time, relaxed and unhurried, to develop a basis of trust. The nurses were asked whether they thought that they had time 'mostly', 'at certain times of the day' or 'rarely' to do so. The option 'not really a nurse's job' was completely ignored. Half (18 respondents) thought that they mostly had time, and a few less that it was only at certain times of the day; only five said 'rarely'. The findings of the observational study (Chapter 4) suggest that they were being over-optimistic.

PARENTS ON THE WARD

Asked specifically whether parents on the ward were 'a help', 'a hindrance' or 'made no difference' to the nurse, everyone (apart from one sister who said they could be a help or a hindrance at any age) thought that they were a help where babies and small children were concerned; with older children they were thought to be either a help or make no difference. Reactions to teenagers' parents were much more mixed: the largest group reckoned that they made no difference, the next that they were helpful, but one in six considered that they were a hindrance. This was despite the fact that the teenagers, who made up a very small proportion of the ward's population, were mostly suffering from cystic fibrosis or were multiply handicapped and had parents who were capable and on good terms with the staff. There was, however, a small group whose problems were thought to be largely psychological in origin and about them there was often a conflict of opinion concerning diagnosis and management. Such cases may have been responsible for the relatively unfavourable view.

Table 6.1 Possible procedures

1. General care of the child	11. Administration of suppositories
2. Temperature taking	12. Administration of enemas
3. Nasogastric tube feeding	13. Monitoring infusions
4. Gastrostomy feeding	14. Taking the apex beat
5. Tracheostomy care	15. MSU
6. Care of indwelling catheters	16. Gastric intubation
7. Post-operative care	17. Wound dressing
8. Physiotherapy	18. Injections as necessary
9. Nasogastric suction	19. Care of chest drains in situ
10. Stoma care	20. Last offices

Three quarters of the respondents thought that parents treated their children in the right way while they were in hospital, although they were inclined to be too indulgent. Some, mainly learners, often thought that they 'don't know what to do' in terms of play and presents.

PARENTS AND NURSING PROCEDURES

In broad terms it can be said that most of these nurses had favourable and accepting attitudes towards parents on the wards, but the crucial question for care-by-parent was how far they thought they could be trusted with the nursing of their children. The topic was introduced in a bland question about whether parents 'might be taught to take over more nursing tasks, particularly for those with chronic conditions'. To this everyone answered 'yes'. They were then asked to consider which of a list of 20 procedures (Table 6.1) most, some or a few parents could be taught to carry out properly, or whether they should be left to those with professional training. Table 6.2 gives the totals for each category of response, but as a few people did not answer every item, n = 710 and not 720; several people omitted 'last offices' for example, either finding it impossible to decide or difficult to contemplate.

Table 6.2 Parents' competence to perform 20 nursing procedures as suggested by 36 Cardiff nurses

	n	%
Parents could do:		
Most procedures	225	31.7
Some procedures	204	28.7
A few procedures	142	20.0
Professionals only	139	19.6
n	710	100.0

Table 6.3 Opinions about parents' competence to perform nursing procedures

	Nottingham: Nurses and SHOs (n = 54)	Cardiff: Nurses (n = 36)	
Procedure	Average parents (%)	Most parents (%)	Professional only (%)
Temperature	22	86	–
Enema	2	42	17
Monitor infusion	2	11	39
MSU	37	65	18
Wound dressing	4	14	31
Injection	2	6	22

Individuals varied from those who considered that 'most' parents could carry out 18 of the 20 procedures and that only one must always be left to professionals (care of chest drains in situ), to one who thought that there was nothing that 'most' parents could be trusted to do. There were half a dozen who thought that everything on the list was possible for at least a few parents.

A somewhat similar exercise was carried out in Nottingham at about the same time (Webb et al 1985), comparing what parents did or thought they could do with what staff (paediatric nurses and SHOs) considered that an average parent was capable of. Many of the things on the list are done more or less routinely by parents in the University Hospital of Wales, and there are only six items on both lists. Table 6.3 compares opinions in the two hospitals on the six common items. Webb et al seem to suggest a low opinion of parents' abilities; for example, only 20% of staff in their study thought that an average parent could give oral medication, while in Cardiff only the peculiarly incompetent did not. However, Webb's figures show that over half the parents were already doing it and that 80% thought that they could. In 11 items on the list, a higher percentage of parents had already done things (obviously a proportion of those whose child required them rather than of the total) than staff thought would be capable. The Cardiff nurses believed that parents were more capable on every item than did nurses in Nottingham. The policy pursued for many years by Mai Davies as Ward Sister and Nursing Officer in Cardiff (Chapter 3) has obviously influenced the thinking of her staff; indeed, the longer staff had worked in the unit, the higher their opinions of parents' competence. The Cardiff figure for monitoring infusions is surprisingly low, since nearly every child on intravenous fluid was monitored by a parent, meticulously. Those who thought they should not were mainly the most recently qualified nurses, all but one of whom chose 'professionals only' for this item.

ATTITUDES TO CARE-BY-PARENT

These findings suggested that the climate of nursing opinion in UHW would be favourable to setting up a Care-by-Parent Scheme, but systematic evidence about the reality and how it worked was not collected on the same scale as for parents.

Sainsbury et al (1986) looked at a series of 32 consecutive children in the CBP scheme and asked the ward sister and the designated nurse for their judgements on the parents' performance and the effects of the scheme on their own role. The main operational problem was the short stay of the majority of patients (suitable for care-by-parent because they were not desperately ill), but by the time participation had been offered and accepted, and the teaching begun, they were often ready for discharge. The option was not offered to two parents who were thought not sufficiently able, and one of the 32 was withdrawn for the same reason. The nurses:

> believed that their relationships with the parents were better than in the traditional method and enjoyed their teaching and supervisory roles in 30 out of the 32 cases. They found it was not difficult to teach the parents the skills required.

This finding is encouraging because it has sometimes been found that nurses feel threatened by the presence of knowledgeable parents. As long ago as 1967, when the point was investigated by Seidl (1969) in Buffalo, New York State, it appeared that while the most senior nurses favoured parental participation, it was least acceptable to those who did the hands-on nursing. Much more recently in France, Brossat and Pinell (1990) found that there could be a hostile reaction from staff to the support that knowledgeable parents could give each other, which is generally regarded as one of the strengths of care-by-parent. The main complaint from the Cardiff nurses in this series was the lack of time to teach parents at the appropriate moment.

The observers recorded nurses' comments about the scheme and their impressions of the way they saw it working. Anyone who had questions was encouraged to ask the author about it, and one of those who did so in the first week was a nursing auxiliary. Her queries supported Sister Carol Eden's contention that insufficient time had been spent in teaching the staff on the wards about the principles of care-by-parent and its implications for their work. The auxiliary had heard a lot but she did not feel that she understood it. After discussing it, she thought it was a good idea, but did not think that mothers should pass nasogastric tubes as it was too dangerous. She was evidently unaware that many mothers had been taught to do this long before CBP, another example of staff not realising what already happens. Parents went home with their babies, intending to tube feed as they had in hospital, only to find that the tubes were constantly coughed, sneezed or pulled out, and, rather than making innumerable return trips to the hospital, they learned instead to pass the tubes. Older children sometimes learned to do it for themselves.

It had been feared that parents would not notice rising temperatures or a deteriorating condition, but Mai Davies was able to assure the 1985 Nursing Times International Child Health Conference that it had never happened with the first 150 parents in the scheme; on the contrary, no change, however small, escaped their notice. Nor did they panic when there was a change for the worse, which had been another worry: they were anxious but reassured by the constant availability of professional back-up. If things got too bad, the nurses could take charge again, which happened once during the observation period when a boy with hydrocephalus developed an ear infection.

Examples of confusion over who was doing what have already been reported. These arose particularly at night, and one observer was told confidently by a staff nurse that CBP did not operate at night, but that the nurses took over again. Another night, at about 10.30 p.m., a different staff nurse was heard to say to an auxiliary, 'Check with Andrew's mother whether she wants to do the observations', but the reply was, 'I've already done them.' Day and night staff now rotate but did not at that time. On the other hand, the CBP nurses were observed to spend considerable periods trying to establish rapport with nervous mothers. One mother, who was reluctant to take over doing anything in hospital, told the interviewer at the follow-up that she had bought a thermometer and used it at home when she thought it necessary, so the time was not wholly wasted. Some nurses commented that it was difficult to run the two systems, conventional nursing and care-by-parent, side by side, since those in the Care-by-Parent Scheme were all at different stages of knowledge and responsibility. A few suggested that a separate unit would be a better idea.

CRITICISMS OF THE SCHEME

At 7.45 a.m. on one particular day, an SEN was with Sean, who was crying, and said somewhat disapprovingly to the observer, 'He is supposed to be a "total care" baby' (not a phrase normally used in relation to CBP). She went on to criticise mothers who 'lie there like a corpse' while their babies cry: 'they think that they will just rest up and let the nurses do it', and implied that this was a problem with care-by-parent. It meant that the mothers were neglecting their responsibilities and the staff were having to cover for them. At that time of day, she might have been on night duty herself and just about to go off, or on days and just come on, but it was a sincerely held opinion, which might easily influence others. Was it a soundly based opinion or an impression, perhaps misleading?

First, in regard to the particular occasion, the records show that Sean's mother said, in passing, that she had fed him at 5.30 a.m., and he was recorded asleep at 6.50 a.m. At 7.20 a.m. his mother was seen walking him up and down the corridor, presumably hoping that she could get him back to sleep. At some point, she put him down in his cot and herself went into the corridor just outside the ward. At 7.45 a.m. he was awake and crying (and the SEN was being critical); at 7.50 a.m. the mother was nursing Sean in the parents' sitting room. She can scarcely be accused of neglecting him.

Second, it is suggested that absent or sleeping mothers were a frequent problem in CBP. Activity sampling shows that babies in CBP were very seldom left to cry alone during the day between 6.15 a.m. and 11.30 p.m. There are no records of the 11.30 p.m. to 6.15 a.m. period, but at the time of this episode the scheme had only been running for 11 nights, so that unrousable parents can scarcely have been a constant difficulty. The nursing officer considered that only someone who was utterly exhausted and in need of respite could possibly sleep through their baby's cries in a cot an arm's length away. The author shares this opinion, and at least one mother was seen to start up out of her sleep when somebody else's baby cried, but no doubt there are some individuals who can sleep through anything.

The nurse's use of the term 'total care' suggests that she may have been thinking of some other experiment in parental involvement, and she also gave the impression that the child should not have been left for a moment. At 7.45 a.m. the mother could easily have been having her breakfast, and ensuring that parents got adequate breaks was part of the philosophy of care-by-parent.

Another night-time problem was day staff suggesting that night care should be left to the nurses, so that a desperately tired mother could sleep, but the message not reaching the right member of staff. At this early stage there was no efficient documentation of the degree of parental involvement or temporary readjustments. Richard's mother complained on one occasion that she had been advised to get more rest and that the nurses would feed her jaundiced baby, but when she woke she found that he had not been fed. Primary nursing would have been an advantage in this instance.

It would seem that the particular SEN's attitude, not antagonistic to the idea of care-by-parent but feeling that parents were not sufficiently committed to it, reflected general ideas based, as least in part, on other experience. There may have been others with similar misapprehensions, who might conclude that effort put into trying to make the scheme work was wasted.

Some criticisms tacked on the CBP scheme really referred to other things: very young mothers were often criticised as being inadequate, and the young mothers in the case studies felt that at least some nurses were unsympathetic. There was disapproval of mothers who left their children to cry, which seldom happened to CBP children. For some mothers it was normal child-rearing practice and, having been told to treat their children as naturally as possible, did what they did at home, however much nurses, doctors and researchers might deplore it. Good child-rearing practice is something which can be encouraged through care-by-parent, but a whole new approach cannot be absorbed in a few days.

On the other hand, the researchers were impressed by the fact that there was no stereotype of the suitable parent. Those who took part in the scheme ranged from the well-educated and affluent to those who were unskilled, unemployed and unsupported.

A NOTE ON DOCTORS

For the most part, the doctors on the wards noticed very little difference – treatment was being carried out and observations recorded. There were some, indeed, who were not aware that anything was happening. They were used to seeing parents there at all hours of the day and night and discussing findings and their implications with them. There was some suggestion that parents in CBP were better informed, so that talking to them was more beneficial to both sides.

CBP AND JOB SATISFACTION

An undergraduate dissertation (Saunders 1985), necessarily limited in scope, looked at attitudes to the Care-by-Parent Scheme and job satisfaction among the nurses. A self-fill questionnaire was addressed to all (114) who had worked on the paediatric unit in the previous year. In a 51% response, nearly all the responses came from learners, which meant that problems of management were not dealt with. The reason for this bias may have been that nearly all the permanent staff had completed the present author's questionnaire and either saw this 'as more of the same' or as a student's project directed at students. Two-thirds of the respondents had worked on the wards where CBP operated, two out of the three wards on the unit, as would be expected.

Both groups of staff (CBP and NCBP) were satisfied with their jobs, the hours and shifts they worked and the status accorded to nursing. Asked about the kind of wards they liked working in, about four out of five included paediatrics among their first three choices. The major dissatisfactions expressed were with the value given to their work by the medical staff and their relationships with senior staff and management, although the CBP group were happier on the last point than the rest. Nine out of 10 who had worked with the scheme enjoyed it, and the great majority thought that it would add interest to their work. Table 6.4 (p.92) is taken from the dissertation and shows that in responses to questions about CBP, there was no significant difference in the attitudes of the two groups, although the NCBP group were more likely to worry that parents would forget something. Both thought that checks by staff should be built into the system.

Comments were invited about feelings towards CBP, and many suggested that parents must be carefully selected and supervised. Its value to the child with a chronic illness was recognised, but many of the points raised could refer to any resident parent or one involved in any way, not necessarily in

Table 6.4 The majority responses to the care-by-parent questions

Question	CBP	NCBP
Worry parents would not carry out observations etc. properly?	No	No
Worry parents would forget to chart observations or carry out a treatment?	No	Yes
Worry parents would not chart an observation accurately?	No	No
Check that parents had done the necessary procedures correctly?	Yes	Yes
Believe the scheme should include nurses' checks?	Yes	Yes
Enjoy working within the scheme?	Yes	Yes
Scheme add interest to your work?	Yes	Yes
Scheme take anything away from your job?	No	No
Scheme a threat to your job?	No	No
Do you think it helps a child to get better quickly?	Yes	Yes
Do you think it helps a parent to cope with future illnesses?	Yes	Yes
Would you like to see the scheme continued?	Yes	Yes
Would you like to work within the scheme (again)?	Yes	Yes
Do you think that a separate CBP unit could work?	Yes	Yes

From Saunders (1985)

CBP. One nurse said:

> I object to drugs being given by the parent as I think it is dangerous, even though they are checked by a qualified nurse.

In fact, this was normal practice with oral medication for any parent who was present and wanted to do it. There was one nurse who worried that learners would lose opportunities to work with some children if their parents were doing the nursing care, a worry shared by some senior nurses beforehand. In the event, CBP children were always the minority, and it did not prove to be a problem. Two respondents made hostile comments, which reflected the professionals' reluctance to share knowledge with the lay person:

> CBP takes away the status of the nurse and makes a mockery of her training.

Comments like this, and the other worries expressed, confirm the tendency for the junior, less experienced, staff to have the most doubts about the abilities of parents and the idea of sharing responsibility with them.

PUBLICITY

After the scheme had been described at paediatric nursing and medical conferences, a great deal of interest in it was shown by other hospitals and by the press and television. A staff nurse was quoted in the *Daily Express* (30.6.86) as saying:

> I think the scheme is excellent because the children are better for it and they are not so scared while they are in hospital. The parents are marvellous. It takes a lot of courage, especially if they haven't nursed before.

A sister, in a feature which appeared in *The Guardian* (25.11.85), said:

> We teach parents everything, however complicated.

Talking to the *Daily Mail* (22.3.86), Sister Carol Eden said:

> This is not really a new role for us, more an extension of an existing one – we already teach student nurses, don't forget.

Sister Carole Davies spoke to Gillian Mercer in *The Independent* (12.5.87):

> The children have somebody they know and love doing things to them. In the past we used to take over and care all revolved around the parents. Now it includes them.

Mai Davies, also in the *Daily Express* (30.6.86), commented:

> Mothers, fathers and grandmothers completely take over . . . Rather than watch someone else injecting their child, parents would rather do it themselves. And mothers don't make mistakes, because it is their own child. We . . . don't make anyone feel guilty if they would rather not take part, but with those who do, it means that there are fewer readmissions to hospital because the parents are also trained to cope at home.

However, by this period, late 1985 to early 1986, the numbers in the scheme had begun to fall and Lee (see Chapter 5) had difficulty in finding a large enough number for her study. Dr Clive Sainsbury, then senior registrar at UHW, who had always taken an active part in the scheme, wrote to the Steering Committee to express his doubts:

> The Care-by-Parent Scheme has been in operation since the summer of 1984. After the initial flurry of activity it settled down to play really rather a minor role in the Paediatric North Ward and almost no role in Paediatric Central. This is despite the genuine belief by those involved with the scheme that it is beneficial, with major nationwide publicity, and almost universal approval. Why is it, therefore, that it has not become a more dominant feature in the wards?

He went on to develop ideas about grades of participation, which he has introduced since at Torbay General Hospital and which were adopted by Chris Bromley in UHW. The appointment of a specialist sister was really the next stage in Cardiff and the following chapter describes her work.

REFERENCES

Brossat S & Pinell P (1990) Coping with parents. *Sociology of Health and Illness*, **12**: 69–86.

Sainsbury CPQ, Gray OP, Cleary J, Davies MM & Rowlandson P (1986) Care by parents of their children in hospital. *Archives of Disease in Childhood*, **61**: 612–15.

Saunders JM (1985) *Study of Nurses' Attitudes Towards a Care by Parent Unit in the Paediatric Department at the Heath Hospital, Cardiff*. Undergraduate Dissertation, University of Wales Institute of Science and Technology.

Seidl FW (1969) Paediatric nursing personnel and parent participation: a study in attitudes. *Nursing Research*, **18**: 40–4.

Webb N, Hull D & Madeley R (1985) Care by parents in hospital. *British Medical Journal*, **291**: 176–7.

FURTHER READING

Carpenter S (1980) Observations of mothers living on a paediatric unit. *Journal of Maternal and Child Health*, **5**: 368–73.

Cartwright A (1964) *Human Relations and Hospital Care*. London: Routledge & Kegan Paul.

Muller DJ, Harris PJ & Wattley L (1986) *Nursing Children: Psychology, Research and Practice*. London: Harper & Row.

7

Developments in the Cardiff Care-by-Parent Scheme

Chris Bromley

When the observation and interview phases of the research project finished in the autumn of 1984, the Care-by-Parent Scheme was running well. However, a combination of job changes, the absence of the research team – whose presence had been a daily reminder – and the fact that the scheme had no formal documentary existence at that time, meant that its operation began to falter. No longer in the forefront of everyone's mind, the opportunity to join in care-by-parent was not offered consistently. The fading out of an innovation, even one as successful as this, is a not uncommon pattern in institutions, as people tend to go back to the old ways.

It seemed clear that someone with specific responsibility for the scheme was needed, and efforts were made to get the funding for a sister who would be in charge. These were finally successful, and Chris Bromley was appointed early in 1988. What follows is her account of how she tackled the job; sadly, circumstances beyond her control meant that she had to leave the area the following year.

For the new start, a new name was chosen – CAPS – Cardiff Assisting Parents Scheme (nurses assisting parents rather than the other way round), and a new logo and pamphlet were devised.

The success of the movement towards involving parents in the care of their children while they are in hospital can be measured by the fact that the scheme did not seem so much of an innovation to Chris Bromley as it did to nurses, doctors, and statutory and funding bodies at the beginning of the 1980s, when the CBP Scheme was being set up. (JC)

BACKGROUND

The publication of the Platt Report on the Welfare of Children in Hospital in 1959 and the subsequent adoption of its recommendations by the then Ministry of Health, marked the beginnings of change in the nursing of children in hospital. The principle that 'children have a right to the care and comfort of their parents' has been the basis of several government recommendations, and the factors central to them are:

1. unrestricted access;
2. the provision of overnight accommodation for parents;
3. the grouping together of children to maximise use of facilities and staff.

Over the last 10 to 15 years, parents have been increasingly involved in the ambulatory care of their children in hospital. Rosemary Thornes (1988) summarises the current situation by stating:

> Parents provide not only security, continuity and support, but undertake many nursing tasks. The system has evolved to satisfy several needs: the child's psychosocial needs; the parent's own need to be usefully employed and to retain some control over the situation; and the system's need for competent parents to continue the care after discharge.

Paediatric nurses have been at the centre of this development and have adapted their working methods to meet the situation. Nowadays, they support, advise and teach just as much as performing traditional nursing care.

The nursing and medical staff of the Department of Child Health at the University Hospital of Wales in Cardiff believe in the philosophy of promoting family-centred care and work together towards that aim. The paediatric unit has, since it opened in 1972, practised unrestricted visiting and welcomed one adult to be resident with any child. Usually a mother or father stays, but a grandparent or aunt may, if that seems appropriate. When parents are present, the nursing staff expect that they will continue to meet their child's personal care needs and feeding unless there are clinical contraindications.

Clay (1986) has pointed out that the nursing profession has traditionally been at the receiving end of change, perhaps arising from 'fear of the new and its reluctance to experiment and take risks'. Despite this conservative tendency, when the setting up of a Care-by-Parent Scheme was suggested in 1981, the reaction was positive, and it was seen by some of the senior nursing staff as the next logical step rather than an unwelcome innovation. Professor Peter Gray (then head of the Department of Child Health) and Miss Mai Davies (Nursing Officer, Paediatrics) had been influenced by the success of American and Canadian units, like those in Indiana (Green & Green 1977), Kentucky (Lerner et al 1972), Vancouver (Robinson & Clarke 1980) and Toronto, which Miss Davies had seen for herself.

The North American units generally had separate premises and separate staff, but in Cardiff the situation was very different because neither of these facilities, nor separate funding, was available: the principle of care-by-parent had to work within the existing establishment and budget of the paediatric unit. The research had shown that it was feasible within the NHS. Two of the three wards on the unit were particularly suitable because one consisted largely, and the other entirely, of cubicles (see Chapter 3). A parents' lounge, kitchen, bathroom and toilet are situated within the unit, and parents could have use of the washing machine and tumble dryer.

DEVELOPMENTS SINCE THE 1984 RESEARCH PROJECT

Following the evaluation of the Care-by-Parent Scheme in Cardiff, the lessons learnt tended to be forgotten in the ever-increasing demands of nursing acutely ill children. Sainsbury et al (1986) reported that:

> A Care-by-Parent option was introduced into a general paediatric ward without any additional finance or facilities. Most parents coped successfully and were grateful for the opportunity of caring for their own children. All believed that their children benefited from their active involvement. The nurses believe that their role was enhanced and their job satisfaction increased. This system offers advantages and could become more generally used by paediatric wards in Britain.

But success was followed by decline, and areas of difficulty had to be identified. In order to make the system operate consistently, it had to be more formal in its organisation, with clearly defined systems for introducing the concept to parents, monitoring its working and providing essential support for the parents.

I was appointed as paediatric sister 'to instigate and manage Care-by-Parent' at the University Hospital of Wales in April 1988, without any ward-based responsibilities and with the earlier experiences as my pointers to methods of rekindling interest and making a workable scheme. In order to re-establish the scheme, parental involvement had to be introduced in a more formal manner and the designated nurse be responsible for the scheme at all times.

It was clear from the first that the nurses on the paediatric wards had actively encouraged parental involvement in care, including teaching parents nursing skills, usually how to record an axillary or oral temperature reading, or how to complete the appropriate column of a feed chart. Although this is good practice, no evidence of parental involvement was incorporated in the nursing care plans.

The first priority was to establish what the nursing staff understood of a scheme that assisted parents to be, in some cases, the primary care givers. At unit sisters' meetings, proposals that would make the scheme effective were outlined and guidelines were provided on what it was considered, on the basis of experience and professional judgement of the group of paediatric sisters, all care that parents might need or wish to be taught. Informal discussions were held to allow staff to air their views and ask questions about how the work would affect them as individual practitioners. It was also the aim to clarify the principles of care-by-parent. There was general agreement that care-by-parent must be encouraged.

GUIDELINES FOR THE SCHEME

Emergency admissions

As the biggest percentage of admissions to the wards involved were emergency admissions, it was felt that any discussion of the scheme would be less threatening to parents if it took place after the family unit had had time to come to terms with the admission to hospital.

Admission procedure

When a child is admitted to the ward, there is a 'formal admission' when a nurse collects important information on the child's normal activities, needs and preferences. It is at this time that parents may express a desire to be resident with their child. This wish should be pre-empted by telling parents right at the beginning that they are welcome to stay and that their presence will benefit their child. However, not all parents will be able to stay with their child in hospital, and some may not want to. As the intention is to offer an individual service to clients, forming a partnership in care which suits the parents' wishes and commitments, this is the time to introduce the concept of a care-by-parent option and to tell parents that if they wish to do so, the nurses will help them later on to care for their own child while in hospital.

First opportunity

An emergency admission is a traumatic experience for all parents. Their concept of hospital is as a place which offers a more specialist service than their GP can provide, and therefore means that their child is very ill. Parents need time to come to terms with what the hospital admission means. The ideal is perhaps for an experienced paediatric nurse to discuss the Care-by-Parent Scheme with the parents after their first night's stay in hospital, but this should always depend on the degree of parental anxiety. Parents should be offered the opportunity of performing all the care they are able and wish to perform. Therefore, discussion between parents and the nurse will have to identify what care parents would like to perform in the early stages. As the admission progresses they will have the option of learning new skills.

Elective admission to hospital

A planned admission to hospital provides the ideal opportunity to prepare both the child and his parents for all aspects of the admission, including participation in care-by-parent.

DOCUMENTING PROPOSED PARTNERSHIP IN CARE

It should not be assumed that all parents will have the same understanding or degree of commitment, and the interests of the patients/clients must always be paramount. The UKCC's Code of Professional Conduct (1984) states:

> Each registered nurse . . . in the exercise of professional accountability shall . . .
> (2) ensure that no action or omission on his/her part or within his/her sphere or influence is detrimental to the condition or safety of patients/clients.

Thus, parents must not be allowed to proceed by themselves until the nursing staff are confident about their abilities. The essence of a care-by-parent option is a flexible relationship between nurses as professionals and the assumption of responsibility for nursing procedures by parents. All parents involved must be monitored, assessed and constantly supported and encouraged. Nursing staff must always be prompt in returning to show parents a new skill or reinforce the teaching already given, never leaving them in a state of indecision about what they should be doing. A daily plan which identifies specific aims for each day should be worked out with the parents. It should specify what can realistically be expected each day and list the observations to be made, specimens to be obtained and treatments to be carried out. With greater confidence, the parents may wish to increase their input of care, but changes in their child's clinical condition, or in their own personal circumstances or anxieties, may mean that they opt out.

A written record in the form of a care plan, specifically with parental involvement in mind, was designed, and this was to be left at the bedside so that both nursing staff and parents could add their comments or achievements. The care plan had also to identify the times at which a parent might wish to hand over full care to the nursing staff – at night, for example – so that the carer could get some undisturbed rest. To make documentation as simple as possible, four levels of care that a parent could perform were chosen:

Grade 1 General Child Care
Attending to basic needs (common to all parents)

Grade 2 Basic Nursing 1 – as care plan 1 plus Charting activities of feeding, nappy changes etc.

Grade 3 Basic Nursing 2 – as 1 & 2 plus Charting observations and collecting specimens

Grade 4 Advanced Nursing includes:

Feeding by:	nasogastric tube
	gastrostomy
	intravenous infusion
Treatments:	giving nebulised medications
	topical therapy
	physiotherapy
	oral nasopharyngeal suction

The care plans, at that time, were arranged under 11 general headings:

1. General hygiene.
2. Elimination.
3. Diet and fluids.
4. General supervision.
5. Parental breaks.
6. Anxieties or worries.
7. Maintaining fluid balance charts.
8. Weight.
9. Specimen collection.
10. Temperature, pulse and respiration.
11. Medication.

The first three aspects concerned most visiting or resident parents whose children were being fed orally, and the next three all parents (but would not form part of a specific care plan), while the rest were mainly for those who were taking on care-by-parent. Two examples (with fictitious names), where mothers were very much involved in the nursing care of their children, are given below. The first sets out the initial responsibilities for a child, admitted for the treatment of a chest infection with intravenous antibiotics, who has an ileostomy.

Care plan stage 3

Patient Bethan, aged approximately 10 months.

General hygiene Daily bath and hairwash by mother prior to pre-breakfast postural drainage and physiotherapy.

Elimination Changing nappies and ileostomy bags (or emptying) as at home. Ileostomy bags normally changed every 2 or 3 days – mother will perform this skill. Calamine lotion to be applied to stoma site at each change.

Postural drainage and physiotherapy to be performed by mother prior to breakfast and before bedtime; other treatments to be performed by ward physiotherapist, at times agreed with mother.

Diet and fluids No change in dietary intake from usual home routine. Ensure pancreatic and vitamin supplements prescribed and have a supply on the ward.

General supervision As at home.

Parental breaks Parents' information booklet given and services available explained to mother.

Anxieties and worries Please tell your allocated nurse if you have difficulties with any of the above or worries about your child's general conditions.

Maintaining fluid balance chart Record all intake of food and fluid; measure all ileostomy fluid and record on chart, as taught.

Weight Weigh nude twice weekly. Tuesday and Saturday, prior to breakfast. Check i/c supervising nurse.

Specimen collection n/a.

Temperature, pulse and respiration Mother wishes to take and record axillary temperature, 4 hrly – normal ranges discussed. Will supervising nurse determine with mother when pulse and respiration are to be recorded.

Medication Mother will check with supervising qualified nurse all oral medication normally given at home and administer it to Bethan. All intravenous medication to be administered by nursing staff – mother not yet ready to learn how to administer intravenous medication.

All care agreed between mother and myself: mother will be resident.

Signed: *C. Bromley*

Any changes and teaching undertaken appear in the second section of the care plan, and the second example demonstrates some of these aspects of the system. Sarah, a multiply handicapped infant, was admitted on this occasion for assessment of distress/pain.

Care plan stage 4 – Advanced nursing

Patient Sarah, aged approximately $3\frac{1}{2}$ months.

Date	*Plan*	*Evaluation/Signature*
17.3.89	All care discussed and agreed between mother and myself.	*C Bromley*
	1. Daily bath prior to first morning feed.	
	2. Changing nappies as necessary – as at home.	
	3. Nasogastric feeds as previously taught, changing tubes as necessary. 3 hrly, via size 8FG tube*, to be given slowly over a period of 30 mins. Mother will perform all feeds from 9 a.m. to 12 midnight*.	**Determined by agreement C Bromley*
	7. All nappies weighed to calculate output accurately. Size 2 nappy weight = . Demonstrate how to calculate weight at each nappy change. Mother will undertake this responsibility when she feels confident.	*2 nappy changes performed – accurate weight & fluid estimate Check again with mother 18.3.89.*
	8. Daily nude weight prior to 9 a.m. feed, to check with supervising nurse.	

10. Mother to take and record rectal temperature (unstable control) as often as she feels necessary or condition dictates, under supervision of nurse. Mother will also take and record pulse and respiratory rates.	*Competent ability – as previously taught C Bromley*
11. Mother to check and administer medication normally given at home i/c supervising nurse.	

DAILY MANAGEMENT OF THE THREE WARD AREAS

Each ward's workload and the skills that parents wish to learn will dictate the time spent with parents. I visit each ward at a time that is convenient for the ward team and review with sister or her deputy any parents who wish to be involved or are just curious. When introducing myself to parents, I chat about their child and the worries that led them to hospital, and discuss my job briefly and the value of involving parents in care. I stress that the extent of involvement – as much or as little as they wish – is entirely the parent's choice, and that the staff will assist and supervise whatever a parent wishes to do. Then a care plan can be devised for each child and his family. Parents need rest, too, so they must be encouraged to leave the ward for meals or to go home for short periods. They must never feel that they are expected always to be there and always to give care. If this happens, staff must question and examine their approach.

Communication between the ward sister or her deputy and the nurse allocated to that child is of the essence so that the teaching may continue throughout the admission. What has been taught must always be documented clearly, as must any problems that may have arisen; this must be reviewed daily and parents be given constant support to keep up their confidence. It is noticeable that when parents learn new skills, they feel a great sense of pride and achievement, and they are usually very meticulous in all that they do. The only qualities required of parents who wish to become more involved in the nursing care of their child in hospital are an understanding of English and the motivation to extend their caring role in a sheltered environment. Simple leaflets setting out the details of the new skills provide back-up information and can be re-read at any time. Some examples follow which give an idea of the kind of conditions that parents learned to cope with.

Example 1

A child aged 18 months, who was part of a very healthy family, suffered a convulsion, associated with a fever, which lasted 20 minutes, while at home.

Both parents were taught how to recognise signs of a rising temperature and how to reduce the temperature without making the child shiver. Guidelines were written down for the parents to read and absorb in their own time, after the principles had been taught. They were also taught the normal ranges of axillary temperature, so that they could check with a thermometer when their child felt hot. Obviously they were taught how to read the thermometer, and during the short hospital admission both parents were given the opportunity to take and record axillary temperatures until they felt confident. In view of the length of the fit, they were also taught how to position the child to administer rectal medication when necessary.

Both parents said before discharge that they could cope with a similar episode should it occur again.

Example 2

A young baby born with a very serious cardiac anomaly, which was considered inoperable, was admitted to hospital aged just 2 weeks, with poor feeding and diagnosed to be in heart failure. Much medication was required to alleviate the symptoms. The mother was taught how to feed via a nasogastric tube, as the baby was unable to feed normally without total exhaustion. The baby had many admissions due to symptoms of unresolved cardiac failure, her main problems being the ability to tolerate only small volumes of feed at any one time, suspected cardiac pain and increasing cardiac failure.

On each hospital stay, usually for reassessment of medication, the mother performed all the care, i.e. the normal parental care, managing hygiene and nutrition. The mother had been taught how to pass a nasogastric tube, how to check that the tube was in the stomach (by aspirating the tube and testing the sample with litmus paper) and, of course, feeding safely through the tube. This mother had wished to learn all the nursing observations, including charting all bodily functions, and to give medication, which, incidentally, was prescribed for the times most convenient in the baby's normal routine. She was also taught to give continuous nasogastric feeds overnight, via a special feed pump, and she became confident enough to increase the prescribed diuretics (within prescribed boundaries) when she noted a raised heart and respiratory rate with increasing tiredness. These skills had been learnt during the numerous hospital admissions, and the mother had been taught how to recognise signs of increasing heart failure when performing the nursing observations of temperature, pulse and respiration. All care was obviously supervised by nursing staff, but this mother learned very quickly and was both confident and extremely competent.

As a sad footnote, the baby died at home aged just 5 months, and, although this mother was alone for long periods (the father worked away from home), she felt confident enough to provide the care to allow her baby to die at home. This was entirely her choice, and when she realised that death was near, she rang the ward to ask if they could stay at home. Her GP and health visitor were exceptional and gave all the physical support needed. I admired this mother's strength and courage, especially in meeting all her baby's last needs; nurses cannot offer what she did – an inexhaustible love.

Example 3

It soon became apparent in a baby who had had a difficult birth and produced lots of oral secretions that feeding was a major problem, with persistent choking episodes. The mother was taught initially how to give nasogastric feeds and then, as it was becoming evident that this method of feeding would be more appropriate, she was taught how to pass a nasogastric tube safely, enabling her to take her baby home. The problem became more severe and life-threatening while at home, as the baby choked on aspirated milk between feeds, causing apnoea. The baby's father gave mouth-to-mouth resuscitation to restore breathing.

The baby required a gastrostomy to ease the problem of aspiration of feeds. The operation was followed by a lengthy stay in hospital, to build the parents' confidence in managing the baby before they could go home again. Oral and nasopharyngeal secretions were still excessive and proved to be a problem at times, so the parents were taught to give postural drainage and physiotherapy prior to feeding and to perform oral nasopharyngeal suction whenever they felt it was necessary. These skills were taught over 2 to 3 weeks, but the support and confidence were obviously needed for much longer. The time spent with, and being available to, these parents was of prime importance. Close liaison with the support services in the community paid off. The GP, the district nurse and the health visitor were the key personnel involved, and all visited the ward to talk to staff and parents on numerous occasions before discharge.

The discharge was staggered over several weeks, the baby first going home for a couple of hours, then all day, then the major hurdle of an overnight stay and, lastly, a weekend. Only then was the discharge felt by all concerned, most importantly by the parents, to be complete. The baby was now 5 months old and had spent a considerable portion of its short life in hospital. On the occasions when the baby was at home, the GP and the district nurse were notified for back-up and reassurance; emergency telephone numbers were given to the parents by all parties concerned. The ambulance service was also notified in case of an emergency, because the family lived at some distance from the hospital and, unless specified, all 999 calls went to a different, nearer hospital.

In order that the burden of being primary care giver did not always lie with the mother, the father was taught all the same skills, at his own request. Cardiopulmonary resuscitation was taught by a member of the medical staff using a resuscitation doll. Then, amazingly, the maternal grandparents asked to be taught everything as well, so that the parents could take a break that did not necessitate a hospital admission. There were two other children in the family, both under the age of 4 years.

During hospital stays, either the mother or the maternal grandfather was resident, and both were more than willing to learn how to perform and record all of the nursing observations, including axillary temperature, heart rate (using a stethoscope), respiratory rate (including the normal ranges and effort involved in respiration, i.e. noting any rib or sternal recession) and recording on the feed chart all intake and output. This meant that they were usefully involved in care and increased their confidence in their own abilities. Experienced nurses always had to be primary care givers in hospital, in order to facilitate the teaching and support the family required to deal with a child who had so many nursing needs.

PROBLEMS WITH THE SCHEME

One problem that has proved very time consuming is maintaining communication with the allocated ward nurse responsible for overseeing the child's care as there could be as many as six different nurses over a span of 48 hours. Therefore, it is imperative that each nurse possess the facts about the care that is required and know exactly what the parents have agreed to do, using accurate, detailed care plans.

It also soon became evident that the original care plans devised for Care-by-Parent were not ideal. These were intended to complement the All Wales Nursing Process documentation. In practice, this proved unsatisfactory because it lacked information about the parent's wish to be involved in care and the 'activities of living'. Consequently, a team of paediatric nurses within the South Glamorgan Health Authority are producing a new format. *This was adopted in 1990* (JC).

To improve the documentation, we have used mainly Roper, Logan and Tierney's (1980) Activities of Living model of nursing. By adding components of the care-by-parent plans, it is hoped to have all the information together without duplication or omission of elements of care.

FUTURE DEVELOPMENTS

The staff of one of the three wards involved have shown an interest in introducing primary nursing. The identification of a defined client group to care for, from admission to discharge, the primary nurse being responsible for assessing, planning, delivering and evaluating care, with help from the associate nurse, must be a giant step towards improving the service the nurses can offer. For example, the number of nurses caring for one patient will be reduced. The primary nurse has total authority and autonomy for her patients. I am sure that anyone working in a system of primary nursing would find that care-by-parent can be adopted with few problems, using the primary and associate nurse as facilitators for parent teaching:

> As the nursing profession develops its right to autonomy and to control its own practice, it also increases its responsibilities to be concretely and systemically accountable for its own performance. Each individual member of the nursing profession must take the responsibility for maintaining high standards in individual practice. The profession as a whole also has this responsibility. (Sorenson & Luckman 1979)

A further development is to produce a simple illustrated booklet, showing most of the common skills that parents learn while in hospital, for example recording an axillary temperature or the more complex skills of nasogastric feeding.

The feasibility of producing a short video has also been considered by the unit sisters. It would be shown in the out-patient department, discuss the care-by-parent option, as in the booklet, and show parents performing some of the skills previously mentioned. This project obviously needs more detailed planning and funding before work can begin.

Another very new venture is to have 'coffee and chat' time, a period set aside each day to encourage parents to come together and get to know each other. A nursery nurse or ward nurse is present to give advice if asked for. As a general observation, non-smoking parents rarely left their child's bedside, whereas the parents who smoked left the ward on many occasions, getting to know other resident parents in the smoking area. Although smoking is generally frowned upon in the hospital environment, it does play a big part in helping parents to socialise and perhaps share their anxieties and experiences. If nurses could facilitate socialising between parents, it would be a small step towards 'normalising' the hospital environment.

CONCLUSIONS

Any unit interested in introducing the care-by-parent concept needs to establish what all the professionals involved understand by the term 'care-by-parent'. Practices different from those currently performed, as well as the alterations which will occur in the nurse's role, must be identified.

This chapter describes how a care-by-parent option was re-introduced into wards at the University Hospital of Wales, Cardiff, after the appointment of a Care-by-Parent Sister. Most parents coped successfully and welcomed the opportunity of caring for their own children. The nurses felt that their role was enhanced and job satisfaction increased.

The role of the nurse with responsibility for care-by-parent is to teach, supervise and support the parents. In the initial stages, this requires a great deal of nursing time: to teach the correct way of doing things and recording findings is time consuming and may need to be repeated several times. A learner nurse may find a job simple after many hours of teaching and instruction, but the parent lacks this and, usually also, the nurse's knowledge base. However, parents' motivation in relation to their own child far exceeds that of learner nurses.

In my experience, parents are conscious of the most minor changes in their child's vital signs and will report them all; nothing will be missed and it may then be difficult to reassure them when the importance of these signs has been stressed.

Care-by-parent can be achieved in any ward setting, but only with commitment from the whole multidisciplinary team. It is not without problems: for example, who takes over from the care-by-parent nurse when she is away on holiday? More and more nurses want the autonomy and authority for complete care; perhaps primary nursing will give the answer. Let the change be what we need to improve the service we offer our clients.

REFERENCES

Clay T (1986) Unity for change? *Journal of Advanced Nursing*, **11**: 21–33.

Green M & Green JG (1977) The parent-care pavilion. *Children Today*, **6**(5): 5–8, 36.

Lerner MJ, Haley DS & McVarish D (1972) Hospital care-by-parent: an evaluative look. *Medical Care*, **x**: 430–6.

Robinson GC & Clarke HF (1980) *The Hospital Care of Children*. New York: Oxford University Press.

Roper N, Logan W & Tierney A (1980) *The Elements of Nursing*. Edinburgh: Churchill Livingstone.

Sainsbury CPQ, Gray OP, Cleary J, Davies MM & Rowlandson PH (1986) Care by parents of their children in hospital. *Archives of Disease in Childhood*, **61**: 612–15.

Sorensen KC & Luckman J (1979) *Basic Nursing*, quoted in Buckenham JE & McGrath G (1983) *The Social Reality of Nursing*, p59. Sydney: ADIS Health Science Press.

Thornes R (1988) *Parents Staying Overnight in Hospital with their Children*. London: Caring for Children in the Health Services, c/o NAWCH.

UKCC (1984) *Code of Professional Conduct*, 2nd edn. London: UKCC.

FURTHER READING

Ball M, Glasper A & Yerrell P (1988) How well do we perform? Parents' perceptions of paediatric care. *The Professional Nurse*, **3**(Dec): 115–18.

Campen Y (1988) Breaking new ground. *Nursing Times*, **84**: 22, 38–40.

Fradd E (1988) Primary nursing: achieving new roles. *Nursing Times*, **84**(50): 39–41.

Jolly J (1980) Meeting the special needs of children in hospital. *Senior Nurse*, **8**(4): 6–7.

Pike S (1989) Family participation in the care of central venous lines. *Nursing*, **3**(38): 22–5.

8

The Philosophy of Care-by-Parent and the Curriculum

Imelda Charles-Edwards

The message of the book is that at the heart of paediatric nursing lies a working partnership between family and nurse in the care of the child. If we really believe that this is part of the essence of paediatric nursing, we must infuse the curriculum with this approach to care.

In this chapter I shall review some of the main implications for paediatric nursing curriculum planning of the care-by-parent philosophy. This book is devoted to analysing the effects of special care-by-parent units on children, their families and the staff. It is important to establish here that good paediatric nurse education will prepare the student for practice in partnership with parents, whether this occurs in a care-by-parent unit, a children's ward or a child's home. The partnership philosophy makes the traditional demarcation line between hospital and home less clear cut, and the curriculum planner can feel justified in integrating this ideal into course planning in the confidence that the student will thereby be prepared to work in any setting – home, care-by-parent unit or hospital.

The care-by-parent philosophy holds that children, whether well or ill, are best cared for by their family, and therefore that paediatric nurses 'will be prepared to share their knowledge and skills' (RCN 1990) with the parents and work with them whenever possible. Such a statement of belief brings into clear focus those aspects of practice, research, management and education which are particularly important to paediatric nurses and, therefore, to curriculum planners.

The word 'curriculum', familiar to educationalists, is not always clearly understood by nurse practitioners and managers. Kerr (1968) defined it as 'all the learning which is planned and guided by the school, whether it is carried out in groups or individually, inside or outside the school'. Kerr's definition shows that the curriculum should encompass every planned happening from the student's recruitment to qualification. The limitation of this definition is that it does not specifically take account of that part of the curriculum which is not planned, the 'hidden curriculum' or the sub-culture of a school or college. It is the hidden curriculum which is difficult for planners to control or change yet which does so much to influence whether or not the course succeeds in its aims, one of which will be to equip nurses to work in partnership with parents.

WHAT SORT OF NURSE DO WE NEED?

Casey (1988) defines the nurse's role within the parent–nurse partnership as being to care, teach, support and refer. The following list, although not exhaustive, outlines some of the qualities required by nurses working within this partnership.

1. The nurse needs confidence in her own knowledge and skills in order to work in close proximity and partnership with parents, to share the role of expert with them and to apply the principles of nursing in a flexible and responsive manner.
   This means that she must accept that the traditional professional-to-patient power relationship is potentially replaced by equality.
2. The nurse needs to be prepared to work without the safe framework of routine and hierarchy, and to have the courage not to conform to the accepted sub-culture if this is antipathetic to the philosophy of partnership/care-by-parents.
3. In order to maintain such close relationships with parents as this work demands, the nurse needs a strong personal self-awareness and professional identity.

It will be clear that a consideration of course content alone would not ensure that a student's experience of education within a course would equip her or him to meet the demands listed above. The course planners must also consider the educational process and, with the college as a whole, the hidden curriculum. The unwritten rules, customs and values of the nurse practitioners, teachers and student body may be incompatible with the values held by the nurse who shares her role with parents.

THE PLANNED CURRICULUM

The key issue which must be resolved at the beginning of the planning process is the choice of the nursing and educational/curriculum models. In the same way as nurses use a nursing model to give a framework for practice, curriculum planners use a nursing and a curriculum model to give a framework for a course. All models represent beliefs or philosophical approaches, in this case about nursing and education.

Obviously, the nursing model selected must be compatible with paediatric nursing and the care-by-parent philosophy. The family-centred care model described by Casey (1988) and Casey and Mobbs (1988) is founded upon this very principle. An example of how this model guides course planners is the way in which it clearly identifies what nursing care is and what family care is, the relationship between them, and how parents may participate in and then take over some of the nursing care by learning nursing skills. This helps planners to ensure that the students learn about the nature of 'nursing' and 'parenting' and the difference between them, clarifies for the students their role with regard to parents, and emphasises the importance of teaching skills. This is one example of the many ways in which a nursing model helps planners to focus upon important issues.

The curriculum model chosen as the framework for a course will represent the beliefs about education of the planners and of the institution within which they work. The model will help to define what, how and when the students will be enabled to learn and how their learning will be assessed. Most of the curriculum models now used in nurse education are compatible with devising a course which fosters the qualities necessary for sharing care and responsibility with parents.

The content of a course designed to foster the qualities needed to practise partnership with parents will not be different from that of many other courses, but the emphasis given to topics and the reasons for this emphasis may be different. Where students must share their expertise with others, it is most important that they learn to value nurses and nursing and understand how their own developing competence is at a deeper level than that achieved by the parents. There is a need to make explicit the relevance of other disciplines (such as sociology) to nursing, within both teaching and practice. One of the values of using a nursing model which is made explicit to the students is that they can then develop a clear concept of nursing and an understanding of why related disciplines are important:

> This is what we believe nursing is.
> ↓
> These are the roles that nurses enact.
> ↓
> Therefore, these are the knowledge, skills and attitudes you need to learn.

One of the greatest problems when deciding on course content is that there tends to be too much to fit into the time available, but the decisions about what has to be omitted from the course which are made in this situation must allow students the time and space to develop academically and personally. In a course which is preparing nurses to work within potentially close relationships between the nurse, family and child, personal development and stress management are essential parts of the curriculum.

THE UNPLANNED CURRICULUM

The reader of a curriculum document will be unlikely to see anything referring to the hidden curriculum. However, an individual who listened to a conversation between a group of students, clinical staff or tutors would soon learn some interesting facts about the subculture of the institution. In most colleges of nursing, tutors spend a lot of time attempting to change the hidden curriculum, even if they are not explicitly aware that this is what they are doing. Colleges of nursing have a written statement of their philosophy, but the intentions inherent in this statement may not be enacted in reality. Both clinical and tutorial staff need to examine the subculture of the college and wards to ensure that, among many things, the students experience attitudes which are positive towards parents and value their contribution to the child's care. This extract (Goodwin 1988) exemplifies how ambivalent attitudes to parents can be:

> Why did the nurses seem so resentful of my presence? Why wouldn't they take any notice of what I said? The admission procedure seemed a bit like the third degree.

Melia (1987) identifies two of the unwritten rules learnt by students. These are the need to 'look busy' and that 'talking is not working'. Bond (1986) also describes this busy syndrome, saying:

> there seems to be a sort of work ethic that we must be on the go all the time to be considered really working. Those aspects which obviously demand a relaxed approach, such as explaining things, teaching, counselling . . . are rarely included in the term 'the work'.

The work ethic which enfolds students, even in a children's ward, may be equivocal about the value of play and talking, making students confused about what is really expected of them. Their problem is magnified by fact that they may be unclear about their role, feeling themselves to be superseded by the parents and others such as playleaders. This is particularly true of junior students who make such remarks as 'I had nothing to do. All the children had their parents with them'. They are tacitly recognising that the parents need expert teaching, support, information (the potential list is endless), which they are not yet competent to give.

So we are confronted by the following problems:

1. Does the work ethic within each ward or department encourage activities such as talking, listening and playing? Do the trained nurses, both teachers and clinical staff, acting as role models, show that they value the parents' contribution and demonstrate the skills needed by a nurse who acts as a teacher, counsellor, resource, leader (the list is long) within a philosophy of partnership?
2. What can we do to help junior or inexperienced students who are working on children's wards?

Attitudes lie at the heart of this discussion. Within basic and post-basic education it is possible to help nurses to become aware of their own values by using, for example, value clarification exercises. Standards should be established for the way in which parents are involved in care. Without such self-questioning and evaluation, a care-by-parent philosophy risks becoming a myth and not a reality, and the students will not internalise the values of the philosophy.

THE PROBLEMS PRESENTED BY DIFFERENT COURSES

With the implementation of Project 2000 courses, curriculum planners are confronted with planning the child-care input to the Common Foundation Programme and the Branch Programme. Compared to the traditional post-registration RSCN courses, both groups of students will be inexperienced. The problem of relatively junior nurses may be reduced but not eliminated by their supernumerary status. There are a number of ways in which those planning and implementing Project 2000 courses can help to overcome some of the problems identified above, with the potential to affect the unplanned or hidden curriculum by what is in the planned curriculum.

The management of the students' supernumerary experience demands that the students are adequately supervised and taught. 'Working with' a trained nurse, using her as a role model, is essential. This may pose problems where student/staff ratios are poor, but where this is the case, the environment will be unsuitable for students. Working with a student sounds very easy, but of course it is not. It is possible to argue that using events which occur in a ward or department to teach one student the subtleties of nursing children within a partnership philosophy requires as much skill as giving a lecture to a group of 100 students. Helping a student to perceive and reflect on experience requires a teacher who is able to perceive and reflect herself and who has the knowledge base to relate all this to theoretical principles and research. At the same time, this teacher has to be clinically expert. This has real implications for colleges of nursing and for the work pattern of nurse tutors.

Inexperienced students need to be protected from unreal expectations of their abilities on the part of trained nurses and parents, while at the same time valuing their own contribution and developing their expertise. One of the ways in which this can be achieved is by setting progressive levels of expectation for students. This may be done through an assessment system which is criterion referenced. In other words, the level of expertise expected of a student in the Common Foundation Programme would be set at a lower level than that for a student at later stages in the Child Branch Programme. The students' performance would then be assessed against these criteria. For example, a student may be aware that he or she could not teach parents to care for their child's central line in the expert manner that they see demonstrated by a trained nurse, but a Foundation Programme student may feel achievement in teaching a child how to clean his teeth properly, recognising that he or she is demonstrating developing skills in teaching. A student during the Child Branch Programme might be expected, for example, to teach parents how to clean the mouth of their debilitated, immunosuppressed child.

Student nurses in traditional courses are sometimes allowed to run before they can walk. Project 2000 courses, by insisting that students learn to walk first, can cause particular frustrations in paediatric nursing where students see parents learning, for example, how to care for their child's tracheostomy, from which the junior students are debarred. This may discourage and confuse students considering their own role, thus weakening their motivation; it can only be tackled by an awareness of the problem, alongside good teaching of the theory and practice of nursing.

CONCLUSION

This has been a review of the main implications for paediatric nurse education of the care-by-parent philosophy. It is clear that, whatever our job, whether it be in practice, management, education or research, we all hold responsibility for ensuring that students learn to value and work in partnership with parents, in order to provide the best care for the children.

REFERENCES

Bond M (1986) *Stress and Self-awareness – a Guide for Nurses*. London: Heinemann.
Casey A (1988) A partnership with child and family. *Senior Nurse*, **8**(4): 8–9.
Casey A & Mobbs S (1988) A partnership in practice. *Nursing Times*, **84**(44): 67–8.
Goodwin P (1988) I know you're busy – but . . . *Nursing Times*, **84**(30): 62.
Kerr J (1968) *Changing the Curriculum*. London: University of London Press.
Melia K (1987) *Learning and Working*. London: Tavistock Publications.
RCN (1990) *Standards of Care for Paediatric Nursing*. London: RCN.

9

Parent Care: A US Experience in Indianapolis

Suzanne Goodband with Karen Jennings

It is perhaps pertinent to start by saying that the direct provision of health care to children in hospital in the United States appears to be extremely similar to that in the United Kingdom. The challenge to the expected in Indianapolis does not lie in an overbearing cost culture: although staff are cost aware, it does not seem to be to a greater degree than one would expect of a registered nurse here in the UK. The marked differences are related to:

- the skill mix of the ward team;
- the relationship with insurance companies;
- cultural differences in the population.

In a parent care unit in the US, the skill mix is based on a fully registered nursing staff. Students observe practice within the unit but never take responsibility for direct care.

Utilisation of resources is important to both the hospital and the insurance company. The insurance company is concerned about unexpected variations in the care of individuals, particularly length of stay, and any departure from the norm. Increasingly, they are demonstrating greater interest in the quality of care the patient receives. The interface with the insurance company is not at ward level but through a member of the utilisation team, primarily nurses. The team is responsible for monitoring bed utilisation and variance in expected practice, and for discussing extensions in stays with the company. At ward level, this promotes an awareness of trends in the care and treatment of children with particular conditions and supports the evaluation phase of care planning. Combined with active quality outcome discussions, a strong evaluative culture develops.

Both as a visitor to the parent care unit and as a non-American, one feels

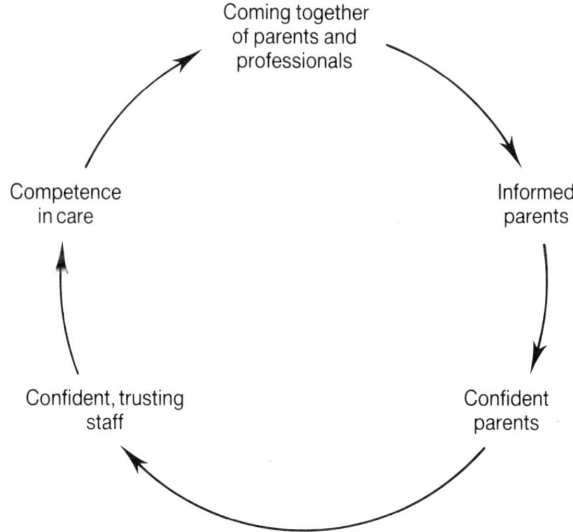

Figure 9.1 The partnership cycle

a strong sense of the impact of the 1960s 'Rights Movement', which appears to empower parents in their quest for equality with the professionals in the care of their sick child. The use of medical terminology, readily, freely and accurately, by parents is both surprising and commonplace. They are comfortable in joining the health-care professionals in the discussions about the child's care and treatment but do not appear to forfeit recognition of their needs as parents of a sick child. It is difficult to assess the impact of these two cultural differences on the development of care-by-parent units. A possible model would be a partnership cycle (Figure 9.1), which relies on the parents and the professionals working confidently together. The parents then inevitably develop a more comprehensive understanding of the child's problems, care and treatment plans, which leads to increased personal confidence. In turn, the staff become more confident in parents' ability to care for the sick child, which communicates trust to the parents and further enhances their competence in care. This leads to parents and staff coming together more and more in the planning, delivery and evaluation of care. When the parents feel confident, competent and key players in the management of the child's health problems, the outcome is the enhancement of the care of the child.

WHAT IS PARENT CARE?

Parent care is a model of care for children in hospital in which the parents retain the responsibility for the care of their children during hospitalisation, albeit with varying degrees of support. It is distinct from the more familiar model of **parent participation**, in which the health-care professional, most commonly the nurse, bears the responsibility for the care of the sick child.

Unfortunately, the two terms have often been used interchangeably, which has resulted in professional staff being unclear about the difference and limiting the opportunity to introduce the concept of parent care more widely.

The development of the two concepts has been quite different in the UK and the US. In the US, they appear to have developed in unison, while in the UK, attention has been directed mainly towards parent participation. However, our observation of practices in the US has encouraged examination of the parent care model.

The James Whitcomb Riley Hospital for Children forms part of a major university hospital and is the only children's hospital in Indianapolis. It both serves the local population and is the referral centre for infants, children and adolescents from throughout Indiana and the Mid-West, with patient care ranging from out-patients through in-patients to maximum intensive care. The philosophy of the hospital is that children need to be hospitalised only if they are seriously ill, require surgery or live far from the hospital and have problems that cannot be managed at home. The staff's belief is that involving parents in educational programmes and in the direct care of their children in hospital will lead to solace and increase their competence as they gain better understanding of the child's health needs. Demystifying both hospital and health care is their explicit goal, so that they can help parents to become effective allies in the promotion of health and the delivery of care to children. British child health professionals share with their American colleagues a commitment to understanding what helps parents and children to cope, as well as increasing awareness of the aspects of hospitalisation which make them weak and vulnerable. Our aim is to develop paediatrics as a parent–child specialty which seeks to strengthen the family rather than leave it powerless and ineffectual.

It makes sense, therefore, to examine a model of care which maintains the parent as the chief observer and best care giver and also offers the parent the opportunity to enhance both competence and subsequent confidence in caring for the sick child. Parent care substantiates and reinforces the role of the parent.

THE DEVELOPMENT OF THE CONCEPT

Post-war research and thinking about the separation of a child from his family stimulated consideration of the situation of the child in hospital. Both the US and the UK responded with increasing parent participation, extending in the US to the recognition that some children and their families could benefit if the parents held greater responsibility.

The work of Burlingham and Freud (e.g. 1942) was the main influence on the staff in Indianapolis, causing them to challenge custom and practice. After confronting what had always been believed to be the best for a child – physical safety above all else – they began to reorganise the principles of caring for the child in any sort of risk into a new order. This order recognised both physical and psychological needs and, in particular, children's vulnerabilities when psychological needs are insufficiently acknowledged.

It became accepted that when children were sick and in hospital, they would probably:

- become more dependent on their parents;
- have difficulty in processing new concepts, particularly the strange, unfamiliar environment,
- have inadequate expressive language and consequent difficulty in communicating.

A parent's presence and access to therapeutic play began to emerge as having paramount importance in retaining some semblance of normality and familiarity.

The early 1960s saw a move away from handing a child over to the hospital for treatment, towards leniency in visiting and residential opportunities for parents. The growing significance of choice in the US during this time meant that children began to wear their own clothes and were offered a selection of food at mealtimes, which was eaten by the bed or in the play/dining room. The long, open ward began to give way to small groups of beds and single cubicles.

During this period a number of chief physicians throughout the US actively promoted shifting the emphasis from treating disease in a child to caring for a child who was sick. The child's need for psychological well-being was acknowledged, and the smaller centres began to follow the precedent set by the large prestigious units.

Health issues cannot be examined in isolation but must be considered alongside other significant changes in the American way of life which have affected the infrastructure of many families. Families became more widely dispersed, leaving themselves with limited access to informal support networks. The increase in the divorce rate and the consequent rise in one-parent families has also reduced the opportunities for informal support. Inevitably, more people became reliant on the formal support of health and social organisations. A health-care response in the early 1970s was the development of two parent care units, one in Kentucky and the other in Indianapolis.

WHAT IS A PARENT CARE UNIT?

Studies undertaken at the James Whitcomb Riley Hospital for Children (Green & Segar 1961, Green 1973) indicated that up to 35% of patient-care days could be spent in parent care facilities. The self-contained unit there, for parents caring for their own children, has six parent care rooms. Designed to look home-like, each has a bed or cot (not of hospital design) for the child, a bed for the parent and en-suite facilities, including a drug cabinet for the child's personal drug supply; internal telephones are provided in each room. The furnishings are also in 'home-style' materials. The unit has a parents' lounge, a nurses' station, a laundry room, a treatment room and a large play/dining area, where parents and children eat together cafeteria-style. Additional juice, tea, coffee, bread, cheese and fruit are available 24 hours a day. The atmosphere is one of privacy, but parents can meet and gain support from each other in the lounge and dining areas.

Providing parent care within a distinct unit ensures consistency in the approach to care for every child. The role of the parent is clear to both families and professionals, which avoids having to begin every interaction by parents reminding staff or staff checking that they are a 'parent care family'. A separate and distinct unit also minimises the risk of comparison and competition between families. The possibility that families for whom this approach may be unsuitable may develop feelings of inadequacy and incompetence should not be underestimated. The separate unit makes the transition from parent participation to parent carer easier and reduces the chance of disappointing other families.

Within a separate unit, it is possible to maintain a calm and peaceful atmosphere, which is conspicuously different for staff who have just left a frantic general ward. To generate a sense of safety for the child and the family, no invasive procedures are carried out in the child's room except for those which must continue after discharge, e.g. insulin injections for the diabetic child.

THE ORGANISATION OF THE UNIT

The unit is staffed by a Unit Director (Head Nurse), two full-time registered nurses and a ward administrator, all of whom are committed to the parent care concept. They have strong clinical backgrounds and are knowledgeable about child development. Ordinary street clothes are worn instead of uniforms. Other key staff groups are 'child life workers' (Thompson & Stanford 1981), housekeeping and dietary staff.

The nursing staff are scheduled on the unit from 7.30 a.m. to 6.00 p.m. Monday to Friday, and 8.00 a.m. to 4.30 p.m. weekends and public holidays. Outside these hours the family may either take the child to the accident and emergency department or call them for advice. Junior medical staff offer the same support to the parent care unit as they would to any other clinical area. However, after the admission 'clerking', a daily appointment schedule, reviewed every 24 hours, is arranged to suit both patient and doctor.

The philosophy of the unit is:

> The parent care unit is a unit where parents live in with their child, assuming 24 hour care responsibilities. Nurses provide education, support and assist with the conduction of diagnostic and treatment plans. Recognising the parents to be the

> most important members of the treatment team, this care facility endeavours to decrease the stress of hospitalisation, promote optimum health care and facilitate family involvement.
>
> Involved are the co-ordinated efforts of all professional workers. It is believed that the term 'parent care' is synonymous with 'parent education' as an integral part of child care. Four important basic elements of care on the unit are: (1) that it is parent- as well as child-orientated; (2) it involves helping the parents with their feelings concerning their child's condition; (3) helping the child with his/her feelings about him/herself; and (4) that it involves education of the parent as part of the treatment of the child. Although we accept the concept that all parents and children need this comprehensive care, this unit provides a unique opportunity for caring for the family as a unit.

The principles of practice in a parent care unit are, therefore:

- the parent assumes 24-hour care responsibility;
- the parent's position within the health-care team is openly acknowledged by all;
- the unit is parent-orientated as well as child-orientated;
- the parent(s) are supported in coming to terms with their own feelings of having a sick child;
- the children are supported in coming to terms with their feelings about themselves and their illness;
- the education of the parent is acknowledged as part of the child's care;
- the environment is both safe and conducive to providing this model of care.

WHO IS SUITABLE FOR CARE-BY-PARENT?

The usual criteria for admission are that the child is not critically ill, the parent is willing to undertake the responsibility, the parent is able to stay, and the physician/surgeon is willing to manage the child's health care within the context of parent care. Each child and family is individually assessed for potential admission to the parent care unit as there is normally a waiting list. The age of the child and the needs of child and the family are considered when establishing priorities. Children can be admitted directly to the unit from home, as transfers from another paediatric clinical area or as transfers from a local hospital.

As a state-wide referral centre, the unit serves a broad range of the child population with complex and psychosocial problems. Children are admitted to the parent care unit with problems as variable as those in a general paediatric ward. Clinical staff believe that children and families can benefit from parent care in the situations listed below.

1. Parents who need to develop skill and self-confidence in administering certain kinds of nursing care or therapy before the child is discharged, e.g. for tracheostomies and gastrostomies, home intra-

venous therapy and the use of equipment such as that for delivering oxygen.

2. Diagnostic evaluations for children with failure to thrive, developmental delay, diarrhoea, vomiting, abdominal pain, neurological seizure disorders, behavioural disorders, orthopaedic and rheumatology problems.
3. Specific feeding problems related to parent–child interactions, breast-feeding anxieties, physical diagnosis (e.g. Pierre Robin syndrome, cleft lip and palate, bronchopulmonary dysplasia, cystic fibrosis and neurological problems), behavioural and psychosocial difficulties, lack of parental nutritional knowledge or environmental deprivation, the transition from gastrostomy to intravenous to nasogastric feed to feeding by mouth.
4. Newly diagnosed diabetes, cystic fibrosis, rheumatoid arthritis or other chronic illness, prior to discharge and in those admitted for reassessment.
5. A child or family needing a home programme of care or counselling from a multidisciplinary team, which includes medical, nursing, dietary, social services and physical and occupational therapies.
6. The over-protective parent, the over-protected child and parent–child separation anxiety.
7. The child receiving daily radiation therapy or chemotherapy if in-patient care is recommended.
8. Short-term surgeries or procedures, e.g. hernia repair, cystoscopy and endoscopy. Some patients may be transferred post-operatively after more complex surgery.
9. When two children in the same family need hospitalisation at the same time.
10. Education and an opportunity to learn care for the parents of infants with multiple congenital handicaps.
11. Transition to home of a premature infant or newborn with long-term problems, e.g. bronchopulmonary dysplasia.
12. Transition between traditional nursing in the hospital and home, e.g. after surgery on a traditional unit.
13. Traumatic amputee or burns patient prior to discharge.
14. Blind or deaf children needing hospitalisation.
15. Selected cases of mothering disabilities or child abuse.
16. Subsequent siblings of infants who died of sudden infant death syndrome or others needing home apnoea monitoring.
17. Patients needing traction, particularly for congenital dislocated hip.
18. Severe constipation, when a child needs initial evaluation and parents need assistance in implementing a bowel programme.
19. Children needing behaviour modification: assistance to parents with their management.

20. The infant or child with cardiac problems who needs continued observation, medication and monitoring of weight gain.

This list is not all inclusive, but it is easy to see that many children admitted to the unit have complex physical and/or social problems, which can be assessed and treated more effectively and efficiently in the parent care setting.

The ability to provide such a comprehensive range of care and treatment raises the question 'When is parent care not suitable?' It is unsuitable if, for any reason, the child is thought to be at risk without 24-hour skilled nursing supervision, if the child requires surgery or intravenous therapy, or if the parents need to leave the hospital.

DAY-TO-DAY PRACTICE

The resident parent (usually the mother) is responsible, with the nurse most familiar with the care programme, for scheduling the child's day. The nursing staff give careful instruction about the child's condition, how to perform skilfully the procedures which meet the child's special needs and how to complete both observation and activity sheets. The parent, with assistance if necessary, can prepare the child for the tests and appointments scheduled for the following day.

Generally, only oral medication is given on the unit, although there are exceptions, such as in diabetes. The nursing staff show the mother how to measure the medicine (kept locked in the drug cabinet in the child's own bathroom) and how to follow the treatment schedule. Parents take children to and from all appointments, such as X-ray and occupational and physiotherapies. They are also responsible for administering all medication (apart from most injections) and recording dietary intake, test and routine observations of temperature, pulse, respiration, bowel activity, etc. The mother's own schedule must allow time for relaxation, consultation with social workers, attendance at parent education sessions and visits to the tea bar and gift shops. Volunteer babysitters are available to watch the child in the parent's absence.

The child's educational needs are met with the support of the hospital teaching staff, and therapeutic play is encouraged and supported by the child life workers.

In parent participation, parents may carry out many, if not all, of these tasks, but it is normally the nurse who retains the responsibility for care and will ask parents what they would like to do in support of the child's care. In parent care, it is the parent who asks for support from the nurse, in areas where he or she feels less confident. Parents initially often feel anxious about clinical support if the child's condition deteriorates (particularly at night) and fire procedures. On admission to the parent care unit, the family is welcomed and told about responsibilities, needs, expectations, unit facilities, policies and fire plans. Attention is drawn specifically to fire exits, extinguishers and the detailed instructions on the back of the room doors.

If a child's condition deteriorates during the day, assistance is available from the unit's nursing staff; during the evenings and at night, the parents can call the accident and emergency staff. The staff on the infant unit will offer direct support when a parent has questions or problems about a newborn infant. Both these clinical areas can be contacted by the telephones in every room, and their staff receive a formal handover and hold the notes and kardex as appropriate.

WHAT ARE THE BENEFITS OF PARENT CARE?

There has been little formal research (until now) into the benefits of parent care, but the clinicians involved in the unit remain convinced by the strength of their daily observations. An endocrinologist, for example, speaks powerfully of how parent care offers a superb opportunity for parents to be educated while their child's diabetes is being controlled. He measures success in the confidence of the parents and their ability to cope after discharge, with a corresponding decrease in telephone calls and emergency room visits. A medical student, opposed to parent care because she believed it indulged and pampered parents too much, has become one of its campaigning advocates since the admission of her own child to hospital. On the general ward, she felt unclear about her role as a parent and primary carer, experiencing feelings of uselessness, isolation and confusion. Transferred to the parent care unit, she soon felt valued and important in the care of her child as she regained some control.

Other parents report how much easier it is to be responsive to their child's particular needs. The mother of an asthmatic child described how she was able to give him his mist treatment at 6.45 a.m., allowing him time to recover his appetite before breakfast. On the general ward, the treatment was given by a respiratory therapist, just before, or even during breakfast, the time determined by the shift pattern and the work load.

In the parent care unit, parents feel welcome and effective, appreciative of the education and, in turn, more able to be responsible for their child's care. They speak of feeling important in the care of their child and feeling good about the positive feedback they receive as they learn new procedures and techniques: this can most succinctly be described as feeling validated. Staff report that as parents become more confident, they become less dependent on formal support, drawing on their own expertise. They become better able to identify when they need help and are less intimidated in requesting it from the professionals.

Many of the staff feel that the non-threatening environment of the unit is an essential component in its success. The individual rooms permit private discussions with social workers and other staff. The decor helps the children to behave more as they would at home, regaining some semblance of normality in their eating and sleeping patterns. The parent's strong position in the health-care team means that the child is less likely to feel abandoned, puzzled or surprised while in hospital.

Parent care gives parents the opportunity to gain understanding of the child's problems over time, rather than in one often hurried conversation just before discharge. They have a chance to think, to check their understanding, to learn procedures and to watch their child's reaction. The family members have time to learn together and to think about how they can manage at home and how they can support each other.

The staff involved in parent care often find that they are asked for support and guidance with everyday issues of child rearing. If family members are experiencing difficulties in their interactions, parent care staff are in a position to appraise the situation and facilitate discussions that may reveal the real aetiology behind a child's behaviour and symptoms.

Students in the various health-care disciplines recognise the unit as a placement where a family-centred approach is required. They report that the 'home-like' setting stimulates the development of the professional–patient relationship; individual children may, in the short term, take up more time, but staff see their colleagues being called less frequently than on a general paediatric ward. They suggest that the hardest part is making the transition from being the 'doer' to being the educator.

THE ECONOMICS OF PARENT CARE

Finance may be one of the key reasons why parent care developed more quickly in the US than in the UK. Studies suggest that parent care is cheaper, requiring less skilled nursing time: Green and Green (1977) refer to average savings of $30 per day in Indianapolis but give no further details.

In Vancouver, Evans and Robinson (1983) compared the cost of providing care on a general paediatric ward with their parent care unit and found the average costs per episode were 33% lower than for general paediatrics, 13.5% lower for tonsil and adenoid surgery and 29% lower for other surgery. Not only was the cost per day less but also the average length of stay was 25% less, which suggests that when the parent is confident, the consultant often discharges earlier. The parent care unit also made fewer calls on the laboratory services. The authors concluded that the greatest savings can be made from the reduced length of stay.

This approach to care can bring economic benefits when resources are scarce but is also justified by the psychosocial benefits it brings to both the child and the family. Could the introduction of parent care units in UK paediatric centres assist in providing a greater quality of care to sick children?

PERSUADING OTHERS IN INDIANAPOLIS

Dr Morris Green, Professor of Paediatrics, and Margaret Martin, Senior Nurse, together gained permission from the hospital management team to promote the philosophy of parent care. They then approached influential members of the community and secured financial commitments to begin a building programme. Having ensured the funds, they turned their attention to persuading the staff involved in the direct care of sick children. An interdisciplinary working party, led by Margaret Martin, set about challenging many established customs and practices until the philosophy evolved.

Having gained the support of the hospital management team, they were able to field the inevitable grumbles and concerns of those keen to protect the status quo. The programme of change began with the identification of a clear philosophy and was followed by a staff development programme for all those who would be affected by the change in approach, including staff in departments such as X-ray and the laboratories. The knowledge and experience of each group formed the base from which to begin their programme. They received formal tuition on the recent findings about child separation and were given the opportunity to consider and challenge the application of the principles to the child in hospital. In the next stage, staff queried the effects that the changes would have on their roles, some of them feeling extremely threatened by the proposals. They raised uncertainties about the safety of the child, the parent's competence and lack of clarity for themselves. Time was allowed for all these discussions and from them developed an understanding about which patients and families would be suitable for this approach.

The interdisciplinary working party considered, at length, the appropriateness of an untrained parent having the degree of responsibility that parent care demands and, deciding where the boundaries should lie, challenged the need for professional control rather than professional guidance in the case of a sick child. The challenge was, first, to gain acceptance and understanding of the concept – that parents could be equals in the provision of health care – and, second, to get permission to try the approach.

In the late 1960s and early 1970s, the staff at Riley Hospital decided to try out the approach; those staff who coached parents and families were rewarded by it, as were those who cared directly for sick children.

The experience in Indianapolis has shown that many professionals benefited from the opportunity to rethink within the safe environment of a development programme and gained from the constant challenge to their ideas. Coupled with the results – seeing is believing – many more of them have come to support this approach, and the education programmes for new hospital staff have ensured continuing commitment.

The opportunity for staff to develop their understanding and resolve problems through education and debate seems to have been the secret of success. However, the commitment and enthusiasm of the pioneers, who were prepared to make a stand for what they believed to be the best for sick children and their families, was what made the change happen in Indianapolis.

WHAT ARE THE OPPORTUNITIES IN THE UK?

Parent care is very different from the usual British hospital approach. It not only enhances the psychosocial care of sick children and their families but also reduces the time the children may spend in hospital, in a manner which has been demonstrated to be cost-effective and, therefore, indirectly benefits many other children. The implementation of parent care allows staff to extend their experience by varying their approach, allows parents the possibility of expanding their responsibilities, to become equal carers of their children, and gives the children a safe, familiar, supportive environment in which they can deal with their own illness.

The benefits were best summarised by Spence (1947) of Newcastle upon Tyne:

> The advantages of the system are fourfold. It is an advantage to the child. It is an advantage to the mother, for to have undergone this experience and to have felt that she has been responsible for her own child's recovery establishes a relationship with her child and confidence in herself which bodes well for the future. It is an advantage to the nurses, who learn much by contact with the best of these women, not only about the handling of a child but about life itself. It is an advantage to the other children on the ward, for whose care more nursing time is liberated. In teaching hospitals it is of further advantage to the students, who gain a practical experience of the form of nursing they will depend on in their practices and learn to recognize the anxieties and courage which bind the mothers to their children during illness: a lesson which fosters the courtesy on which the practice of medicine depends.

ACKNOWLEDGEMENTS

Both authors would like to take this opportunity to thank Margaret Martin and Morris Green for their help in the preparation of this chapter. Suzanne Goodband would also like to acknowledge with thanks the support she received from both the Band Trust and the Florence Nightingale Memorial Committee, which enabled her to visit the parent care unit in Indianapolis.

REFERENCES

Burlingham D & Freud A (1942) *Young Children in Wartime in a Residential War Nursery*. London: George Allen & Unwin, for the New Era.

Evans RG & Robinson GC (1983) An economic study of cost savings on a Care-by-Parent Ward. *Medical Care*, **21**(8): 768–82.

Green M (1973) Innovative methods of expanding ambulatory services. *Advances in Pediatrics*, **20**: 15–38.

Green M & Green JG (1977) The Parent Care Pavilion. *Children Today*, **6**(5): 5–8.
Green M & Segar WE (1961) A new design for patient care and pediatric education in a children's hospital: an interim report. *Pediatrics*, **28**: 825–37.
Spence JC (1947) The care of children in hospital. *British Medical Journal* (i): 125–30.
Thompson R & Stanford J (1981) *Child Life in Hospital: Theory and Practice*. Springfield, Ill: Charles Thomas.

FURTHER READING

Anon (1983) Care-by-parent pediatric hospital services. *Alternative Designs*, (Nov/Dec): 3–7.
Jennings K (1986) Helping them face tomorrow. *Nursing Times*, **82**(4): 33–5.
Jolly J (1981) *The Other Side of Paediatrics*. London: Macmillan Press.
Lerner MJ, Haley JV, Hall DS & McVarish D (1972). Hospital Care-by-Parent: an evaluative look. *Medical Care*, **X**: 430–6.
McMahon L & Goodband S (1990) Making changes happen. In Fielding P & Berman P (eds.), *Surviving in General Management*, pp. 172–184 London: Macmillan Press.
Vermilion BD, Ballantine TVN & Grosfeld JL (1979) The effective use of the Parent Care Unit for infants on the surgical service. *Journal of Pediatric Surgery*, **14**: 321–4.

10

Care-by-Parent – the Basis and the Options

In recent years, there has been a general movement, a change in climate, in work concerned with people who are in some way disabled, towards realising that they have a contribution to make in managing their affairs. Their problem may arise from immaturity, congenital handicap, illness, trauma or the inability to cope with their lives or their responsibilities within the constraints of their environment, be these personal, social or economic.

Previously, the tendency had been to take all control away from those seen as incompetent and to do what was best for them, with the emphasis on physical conditions and controlling behaviour. Decisions were made for them, and their lives were arranged in their own best interests; that the inadequate (and in many fields 'lay' was assumed to mean 'inadequate') might have abilities and useful insights, or that their reasons for action had any validity, was scarcely considered.

Gradually, professionals became aware that their actions were not necessarily producing the desired results, and some lay people were becoming more articulate about their disquiet. In particular, it was recognised that removing people, especially children, from all that was familiar to them produced another kind of displaced person (NISW 1988). Limited intervention in people's lives, in both health and social work, has become the preferred means of altering damaging situations, making use of the resources of the people involved, respecting their values and listening to what they say (Fisher 1983). The aim is now that the professional and the client should work together towards an agreed, acceptable goal which has taken account of the client's point of view. The professional should be a partner rather than a benefactor-cum-despot; independence is the object of the exercise (Clode et al 1987). This new style of relationship is spelled out for children in the new Children Act 1989 (Bridge et al 1990) and was foreshadowed in the Platt Report.

Within paediatric nursing, these changing relationships have become more explicit in recent years. The Children Act (1989) is among the bases of the *Philosophy* for Paediatric Nursing Entities (RCN 1991); the others mentioned are two international declarations on the rights of children – from the UN (1989) and the EEC (1986) – and, from Britain, the NAWCH Charter (1985) and the UKCC Code of Conduct (1984). The *Philosophy* stresses first the need to inform and involve both the child and the family in planning and decision-making for health. The child is to be seen as an individual and as part of a family. Second, it emphasises that the role of the paediatric nurse is to promote, by both proactive and reactive means, the best interests of individual children and children in general and, where needed, to act as their advocate.

These changes are sometimes reckoned to be part of a general consumerist movement, but in the field of health this seems a misleading term, suggesting a level of choice which the patient rarely has. He or she cannot decide what kind of illness will occur (despite Balint 1968) or send back an unsatisfactory operation, and rarely has detailed knowledge about the available options in consultants or treatments or the skill in manipulating the 'gate-keepers' to them. The term 'gate-keeper' is used in sociology to mean someone who controls the lay person's access to certain kinds of professional, particularly those at the higher levels; for instance a patient can see his GP, but cannot make an independent approach to a consultant. The gate-keeper has two main functions: first to protect the professional from ill-judged or frivolous demands (the lay person is often assumed to be incapable of making a sound decision about whether a professional's services are necessary and of what kind these should be); and second, to regulate the workload by controlling the flow of applicants – by exercising power, he or she enhances the status of his or her own group.

Children, as well as being more vulnerable to the institutions and processes involved in treatment, are rarely able to speak or act on their own behalf, although 'listening to the client' is beginning to be extended to the young, for instance see the Children Act (1989) section 1(3) (a). Parents are – in the absence of any evidence to the contrary – considered to be the child's best advocates and it is they who are expected to partner the professionals in the care of sick children. In a few conditions, like diabetes, and some procedures, like intermittent catheterisation and nasogastric intubation, the child, too, may become a partner.

DEVELOPMENTS IN NURSING

Parellel with these changes in attitude to clients and patients, and their place within the health and social services, has been the emergence of nursing as a distinct discipline. Although Florence Nightingale (1859) gave her *Notes on Nursing* the subtitle *What it is and What it is not*, she was concerned to lay down rules and precepts rather than to define, and described them as 'hints for thought to women who have personal charge of the health of others' rather than hospital nurses. Her concern with the airing of rooms, diet and avoiding shocks and irritations – 'the fidget of silk and crinoline . . . the creaking of stays' – reflects the lack of effective pharmaceutical products as well as the fruits of her own experience. However, her opening statement that 'disease . . . is a more or less reparative process' strikes a more contemporary note.

Nursing had developed on a somewhat ad hoc basis, responding to changes in medicine and surgery, tacking traditional practices on to new procedures without much consideration of their necessity. The anomalies which had arisen and the need for appraisal, among other things, stimulated the Royal College of Nursing and the then Ministry of Health to collaborate in setting up, in 1966, a series of research projects, the first to be designed and carried out by nurses, to examine the quality of nursing care and develop appropriate research techniques (McFarlane 1970, Inman 1975). In the same year, Virginia Henderson's (1966) famous definition of nursing was published, which focused on the needs of the 'individual, sick or well' and nursing's function in assisting him to 'gain independence, as rapidly as possible'.

The following year saw the publication of the first edition of *The Nursing Process* (Yura & Walsh 1967), which has profoundly affected the approach to patient care in hospitals where some form of its analytical framework has been adopted. Since then there have been many definitions and bids to provide a sound theoretical base for nursing, most recently in the development of nursing models. These are considered, and their effects on the delivery of appropriate care evaluated, in Kershaw and Salvage (1986) and Salvage and Kershaw (1990). In the latter volume, Glasper (1990) describes how his unit developed its own model for paediatric nursing care and the appropriate documentation which would encourage, if not ensure, its use on the wards. For the nurse on the ward, the forms that are used in recording information about the patient and planning and assessing the care are the outward and visible sign of the theoretical basis for what the nurse is doing. Whether they provide suitable and adequate space to include the parents' actual and potential contribution to care may be crucial to their successful participation. Without it, the nurse, particularly one new to a paediatric ward, may not be reminded of the part that parents can play or be aware of what particular individuals are already capable of doing.

STANDARD SETTING

Another recent movement in nursing has been the setting of standards for care in particular clinical and service areas, which will be reflected in both policy, at hospital and ward level, and the care of the individual patient. For children, the major input from the profession, following on from the *Statement of Values in Paediatric Nursing* (RCN 1987), is *Standards of Care for*

Paediatric Nursing (RCN Paediatric Standards Working Group 1990), produced by a Working Group chaired by Anne MacDonald and part of the RCN Standards of Care Project (Kitson 1989). This was part of the third stage of the work, begun with the research projects of the 1960s and followed by an expert group set up in 1978 which was chaired by Dame Sheila Quinn (RCN 1981). The recent work is producing a series covering various areas of nursing. For paediatric nursing, 20 standards of care for children in hospital are set out, intended to form the basis for locally agreed versions. They must be considered in relation to each other, rather than each being taken as the last word on its own subject.

The standards are set out under five topic headings, each with several sub-topics. The topic headings are:

- Family-centred care.
- Safety.
- Individualised patient care.
- Continuity of care.
- Communication.

For the purpose of this work, the most important element is how far the presence and involvement of parents is integrated into the standards. They do assume throughout that it is in the best interests of children that their parents should be present, involved and informed; significantly, 'family-centred care' is the first topic to be considered.

Each topic begins with a standard statement, a general principle, and under 'Family-centred care' the first subtopic is 'Parental visiting'; its standard statement is 'Parental visiting will be unrestricted for all children in hospital'. It then sets out the requirements for achieving this aim, under the headings 'Structure/Resources' and 'Process/Actions', followed by 'Outcome', which in the case of Standard 1 is simply 'Family links will be maintained'. Each is supported by references. For Standard 2, concerning resident parents, the outcome is in five parts, covering awareness of the right to be resident, parents' contribution to care and staff attitudes to parents, both those who are resident and those who are not. The other subtopics under 'Family-centred care' are:

- Preparation for elective admission.
- Parental involvement in giving care.

The latter is reproduced here (Figure 10.1) as it is most relevant to the subject of this book and because it shows how far professional thinking has gone towards accepting ideas which were considered daringly experimental or just unnecessary when the care-by-parent scheme was being discussed 10 years ago.

The second topic of the Standards of Care document is safety, and parents are mentioned only as people who may escort children to other parts of the

Standard 4
Care group: Children in hospital
Topic: Family-centred care
Subtopic: Parental involvement in giving care
Standard statement: Parents will be encouraged to be actively involved in the care of their child in hospital.

Structure/Resources
1. There will be a Registered Sick Children's Nurse on duty at all times.
2. Ward organisation will allow the practice of individualised patient care.
3. The ward philosophy will encompass parental participation in giving care.
4. All nurses will be prepared to share their knowledge and skills.
5. All children's wards will have facilities that enable parents to participate in giving care.
6. Written information will be available to support and remind parents about specific aspects of care.

Process/Actions
1. On admission, a nurse will negotiate with the parent the degree of parental involvement in giving care.
2. The nurse will assess priorities of care with the family.
3. The nurse will plan care with the parents and child and record it.
4. The nurse will teach the parents any skills required in order to give the care negotiated.
5. The nurse will supervise parents until competence is achieved.
6. The nurse will indicate that she is available to offer support and advice.
7. The nurse and family will evaluate the child's care and reassess priorities as necessary.
8. The nurse will give the parents any specific information leaflets.

Outcome
1. Parents will understand their role in giving care.
2. Nurses will know the extent of parental participation in giving care.
3. The child will receive care from the parents as planned.
4. Parents will feel in control of the care given to their child.
5. The parents and child will be included in the assessment, planning and evaluation of care.
6. Parents will be prepared to provide any ongoing care required following discharge.

Figure 10.1 Parental involvement in giving care

hospital and not in relation to the administration of medicine. The third topic (Standards 11–15) includes parents in planning care, assessing pain and being encouraged to participate in play. Standard 16 (topic 'Continuity of Care'), 'Emergency admission to hospital', also touches upon parental involvement –

being resident and taking part in planning and giving care, both in hospital and after discharge, and the information and education which will be required. Standard 19 is unequivocal about the child's need to be accompanied by a parent in the anaesthetic room, still a contentious issue in some quarters (Glasper & Dewar 1987, NAWCH 1987, Day 1987, Coulson 1988, Glasper 1988, and an RCN Congress resolution 1990).

Standards 14 (topic 'Individualised patient care; subtopic 'System of nursing care') and 20 (topic 'Communication'; subtopic 'Reporting of patient care') enjoin the use of care plans based on an 'appropriate model of nursing care' and handover reports 'by the nurse caring for each child to the nurse taking over the care of the child, preferably on a one-to-one basis', which has implications for the structure of the delivery of nursing care.

Setting standards is the beginning of a process and achieving them should follow, but maintaining them when they require changes in attitude and practice is the most difficult part. Frequent monitoring is necessary to ensure that new standards continue to be observed, a time-consuming and complex business. It involves seeking the opinions of the people on the receiving end of the services. Ball et al (1988) describe a pilot study of parents' perceptions of care in one paediatric unit and speak of the need for units to 'become fully self-evaluating'.

Some of the impetus for formal standard setting and evaluation has come from outside the profession, in the work done by the National Association for the Welfare of Children in Hospital (NAWCH, now known as Action for Sick Children) with the *NAWCH Quality Review: Setting Standards for Children in Health Care* (Hogg 1989), which has developed from their *Charter for Children in Hospital* (1985) and the *Quality Checklist* of 1988. They quote the WHO definition of a standard in health care as 'an agreed level of care required for a particular purpose' which should be 'reasonable, understandable, useful, measurable, observable, achievable'. They have based their standards on guidance from the Department of Health and professional organisations concerned with children, and have adopted wider terms of reference, covering matters of policy and management in both hospital and community, in both proactive and reactive services. After discussing the standards set, the *Quality Checklist* supplies a series of checklists, designed to evaluate most aspects of the child's health care at various levels:

Policy matters:
- DHA
- clinical
- nursing
- preventive
- information and statistics

Service provision:
- in-patient
- out-patient
- A&E department
- diagnostic and support
- paediatric services in the community

Consumer survey instruments

It stresses the need to monitor practice and revise and update the standards as becomes necessary or possible.

The information collected can 'be drawn together to provide an overall profile of services for children' and to look for discrepancies in the replies from various staff groups or between staff and parents; either may indicate areas where policy change is needed or practice should be reviewed. Questions about the role of parents (perhaps surprisingly) play a relatively minor part and relate mainly to normal personal care, although 'treatment' and 'administration of medicines' receive a mention.

The nursing process, nursing models and standard setting, perhaps a widespread move towards primary nursing and all the changes that that would imply (Fradd 1988), are all factors in the rapid development of nursing which will profoundly affect the way in which children and adults are nursed. Their evaluation and selection among them is the province of the members of the profession, but the author would, nevertheless, like to comment on some aspects of these prescriptions for improvement: first, to welcome the emphasis on the knowledge of child development in the RCN document *Standards of Care for Paediatric Nursing*; second, to express the hope that sufficient resources will be available to produce, marshall and update the documentation required (care plans, including some for particular conditions, pre-admission booklets, parents' leaflets on conditions and procedures for use on the ward, information to take home and survey instruments in whatever languages the demography may demand); and, third, to stress that the people who have to use them need to be consulted about the form they will take.

Community health services, including domiciliary nursing services, have been outside the scope of this study, but current trends make it seem likely that there could be a whole spectrum of care, from intensive care in hospital, through varying degrees of professional and parental responsibility in the ward, to varying degrees of professional intervention with the sick or recovering child at home, to normal family care, which will always be the base of the pyramid of health care. All this requires efficient liaison and easy communication.

On top of all this comes Project 2000, PREPP and the 1990 NHS Act. Children's wards have aimed at having supernumerary students for many years; Project 2000 should provide a better supply of qualified paediatric nurses and will, at least, remove the fear that care-by-parent will limit learners' opportunities for experience. Will the numbers of experienced qualified staff be sufficient to take on the teaching and support roles needed for participating parents? Will the services of resident parents come to be taken for granted, whatever their circumstances? Will the operation of the internal market under the new Act and the development of specialist centres ensure separate provision for children, recognising their developmental needs and vulnerability? Will facilities for parents and for play be safeguarded or left to the voluntary sector? If community paediatric care is more widely adopted, will there be sufficient resources to provide care and support round the clock? Will respite care be available when it is needed? Will the proportion of children nursed on adult wards and outside paediatric supervision be reduced? Staff might be forgiven for finding the prospects daunting rather than just challenging.

THE WELFARE OF CHILDREN IN HOSPITAL 1991-STYLE

The new Department of Health (1991) publication *Welfare of Children and Young People in Hospital* is not as controversial as its predecessor of 1959. It is described as a guide and reflects the good practice of most hospitals rather than suggesting any revolutionary changes. The Cardinal Principles set out (in Section 2.1) would all fit easily into Platt, although there are no longer references to 'discipline'. There is greater stress on the child's right to information, the special needs of adolescents and ease of access to facilities. The most important aims are the consideration of the whole child and the coordination of the child's care throughout the various parts of the NHS – summed up in the phrase 'a "seamless web" of care, treatment and support' (Section 1.1).

Section 4 deals with the 'special needs' of children and stresses the need for 'complete ease of access to the child by his or her parents and to other members of the family' and 'This is not a luxury. It . . . is fundamental to the care and treatment of children in hospital'. However, the role of the visiting or resident parent is seen mainly as carrying out normal child care and learning clinical procedures 'which will enable them to care for their child at home after discharge' – essentially similar to that described in Platt (1959: para. 69). Service specifications include providing 'maximum help and advice to parents to enable them to play a part in the care of their children and to *continue the care* following the child's discharge from hospital' (emphasis in the original).

No precise guidelines are given on the nature and amount of accommodation to be provided for parents, but the recommendations of *Parents Staying Overnight with their Children in Hospital* (Thornes 1988) are quoted. It is suggested that more facilities will be required than were outlined in *Hospital Accommodation for Children* (Hospital Building Note No 23 1984).

The manner in which life-threatening illness and the death of a child should be approached with the family is considered (Sections 4.38–4.43) – a subject not dealt with in 1959. 'Long-stay hospitals', on the other hand, no longer appear as an important category.

The idea of care-by-parent, that it is desirable that the parent should, whenever possible, take on the nursing care of the child who is *in* hospital, not simply as preparation for discharge and, that this provides optimal care, has not been embraced. It will be the responsibility of forward-looking commissioners and managers to build it, as part of the 'seamless web', into the specifications for children's care.

THE TORBAY SCHEME

In 1986 Clive Sainsbury went to Torbay as consultant paediatrician, and one of his first aims was to start a care-by-parent scheme. He had already seen a tendency to decline in the scheme in Cardiff and formulated ideas about how to make it work more smoothly and acceptably. With the support of unit management, the senior nurses and most of the ward staff, TOPPS (TOrbay Parental Participation Scheme) came into being in November 1987. The main innovations were a nurse with 'protected time' to run it and a system of grades of parental involvement. The unit funded the part-time secondment (for 6 months) of a clinical teacher with responsibility for paediatrics to get the scheme going. She was familiar with the wards and their staff and had proven teaching skills.

When parents joined the scheme, they took over nursing work gradually, and the stage they had reached was indicated by the colour of the care plan (pink, blue, yellow and orange) on the clipboard at the end of the bed. Each stage added on to the ones before. The entry grade comprised normal child care, the next added monitoring and maintaining fluid balance, and only in the third stage did they learn TPR observations, which most were very keen to do. Karen Jeffery, who was running the scheme, was anxious for parents to understand that the purpose was to improve care for the child by limiting the numbers who were involved in it to a familiar few (as few as possible) rather than to relieve the staff of nursing tasks. The majority of parents did not go beyond this level of involvement because the child's condition did not require it and the length of stay did not permit it. The fourth stage was open-ended and could include anything that a seriously or chronically sick child might need; it was reached by those with prolonged admissions. Parents joining the scheme were given a list (Figure 10.2, p. 136) which indicated the kinds of task that most of them would be doing and that they were taking on responsibility for them. This did not appear to put anyone off.

Responsibility for medication can be problematic because of the possible dangers and the legal implications. Ideally, parents who have taken on the responsibility for nursing care should have control of the supply and administration of the child's medication – oral or topical – as they would at home, but it is difficult to provide secure storage within the ward. In Torbay, medication remained with the staff but was administered by parents under the supervision of a qualified nurse; both parent and nurse signed the drug prescription chart. The idea that parents should sign for the procedures they

1. General hygiene: bath, wash, care of teeth, etc.
2. Elimination: nappy changing, toileting.
3. Ensure an adequate diet and fluid intake as at home or as indicated by the doctor.
4. Generally supervise throughout the day as you would at home.
5. Maintaining the fluid balance chart: this means recording all dietary intake and output.
6. Weighing: this is on a regular basis (as required by the doctor) and charted on the chart provided.
7. Taking and recording temperature, pulse and respiration as prescribed.
8. Checking and giving of all medication, with the allocated nurse, as prescribed:
   (a) throughout stay;
   (b) in readiness for discharge.
9. To perform all of the above and more as indicated.

This list is only meant as a guide to those tasks performed by the nurses. If you feel that you wish to participate in the TOPP Scheme and perform *some or all* of these you may do so. Instruction will be given until you feel confident and happy to perform them.

From Jeffery 1987.

Figure 10.2 Parental responsibility

have taken on seems a good one and could usefully be extended to include other items on the care plans. This is already done on some domiciliary nursing schemes, for example in Kettering (Sidey 1990).

Karen Jeffery acted as a coordinator and primary teacher of parents, but each child also had an allocated nurse who reinforced the instruction given and was always available for assistance and reassurance. A self-completion questionnaire for parents indicated that more than three quarters of them knew that they could stay with their child in hospital. As in Cardiff more than half had to make arrangements for other dependants, and many took time off work (Jeffery 1988). The scheme worked successfully for many months, particularly during the secondment, but there has since been some decline in commitment towards it, and it is felt that there is a continuing need for a nurse with specific responsibility for it. New senior staff and new documentation, which lays emphasis on parental involvement in care, may reinvigorate the scheme.

In Southampton, a care-by-parent scheme is running as an option in the new Paediatric Oncology Unit, which opened in the summer of 1991 (Glasper 1992).

WHAT HAS BEEN LEARNED?

This book has covered many aspects of the lives of children in hospital, the history of such care, factors influencing changes in practice and more recent events which have been influenced by conscious attempts to improve the psychosocial rather than the physical aspects of their treatment, as well as the research which has attempted to evaluate this.

It has focused upon the introduction of a care-by-parent scheme to a paediatric unit and has also examined the lives of children conventionally nursed in an open ward. Prolonged observation is a time-consuming and expensive method of gathering data, but without it it would have been difficult to arrive at any comprehensive idea of how children in hospital spend their time. The pattern of life there is very different from life at home and can vary considerably, not only with the age of the child and his or her condition but also with the amount of visiting, the effect of treatment upon mobility, the position of the bed within the ward and the presence or absence of congenial companions. An individual child may be lonely in a room that is never empty, while a clear view of the television set may be familiar and comforting if not exactly entertaining – one morning 'Sesame Street' was turned off during a doctors' round and the set switched on again later when it was showing a test match.

Much of the impetus for change during the 1950s and 1960s came from those whose main concern was the psychological needs of children and particularly the after-effects of hospitalisation; they were, therefore, mainly from outside nursing. The acceptance of unrestricted visiting, resident parents and the role they are expected to play in hospital has developed patchily and piecemeal over the country, and in some areas acceptance has been slow in coming. Gradually, with succeeding generations of nurses, the presence of parents on paediatric and some other wards with a large proportion of child patients has become normal and desirable. In fact, getting used to the idea, so much at variance with previous beliefs, was a large part of what was needed to allow the change to take place. Care-by-parent as a matter of policy, on the other hand, requires more active cooperation by nurses and greater commitment to the idea. It remains to be seen whether changes in the nature of nursing, as a profession and a discipline, with a new educational system leading to a new set-up on the wards and including two distinct classes of worker, will facilitate the development of parental participation and care-by-parent schemes.

PLANNING FOR CARE-BY-PARENT

The author's perspective on this topic is derived from observation, research (over many years) and the literature, and will obviously differ from that of the practising health-care professional; thus, these observations are offered with some diffidence.

The first thing to be said about care-by-parent is that it works, from the point of view of the patient, the parent, the nurse and the doctor. Given the right circumstances, it will be a successful addition to the options in the care of sick children. The difficulty is in preparing the right circumstances and maintaining them – especially in maintaining them. Innovations in hospital often only last as long as the active involvement of the initiators, or when some outside factor, like a research project, adds a touch of excitement to the situation.

THE ESSENTIALS – COMMITMENT AND CONTINUITY

When the author was looking back over the work of the Cardiff scheme, she was struck by a phrase from an article on professionals and parenting (Hooper 1981) which encapsulated what good parents provide as being 'commitment and continuity'. This also sums up what they can offer to their children in hospital, at the time when they are in most need of them, to an extent which is impossible and undesirable for a nurse who has work to do and a life to lead outside it. However, further reflection showed that care-by-parent also requires commitment and continuity from the nursing staff, not to the individual child but to the concept. Without them schemes will falter and decline until they become part of a legendary past, although the occasional parent who has participated before may ask to do so again. Publicity helps to keep the idea going, but it is not enough in itself and may lead to little more than occasional gestures.

It is essential that everybody knows about a care-by-parent scheme, that it becomes part of the whole hospital and not just an odd quirk of a remote unit. Time must be provided to instruct staff in how it works and how they must work with it and to give the concept its due weight. The success of the Indianapolis unit has been maintained by a continuing staff education programme. Commitment is needed from the top down, particularly in the UK where the direct reduction of costs to the family is not a factor which promotes interest in care-by-parent.

APPROACHES TO CARE-BY-PARENT

There are two broad approaches to care-by-parent, which may be called exclusive and inclusive.

The exclusive approach

This is the preferred choice when one of the main aims is cutting costs, which it does by excluding everything that does not fit into the scheduled categories and patterns of working. It has been adopted by some American hospitals in recent years. Admission is to a unit separate from the wards, and using it rather than the main wards is part of the decision to admit, taken before the child arrives at the hospital, although transfers may be possible. Parents may have to choose to go to the unit rather than the ward without much information.

Admission is based on strict criteria of suitability, in Galveston that the child should 'not be acutely ill' and that 'all care on the unit can be provided by the parent' (Caldwell & Lockhart 1981). The unit will have its own 'gate-keepers' whom the admitting doctor will have to convince.

The conditions which are considered appropriate for such care are those whose course is almost entirely predictable. They tend to be investigations, minor surgery, education for, or reassessment of, chronic conditions or even more specific cases, like 'readiness for gait training' as described by Monahan and Schkade (1985) in Dallas. It is the condition, rather than the child, which is significant.

Having restricted entry to the unproblematic, and the parent being responsible for the care, staffing can be minimal. In the Galveston unit, a coordinator is present from 7 a.m. to 11 p.m., but the only nurse who routinely appears on the unit is the night supervisor who includes the unit in her rounds. This is the extreme form of the scheme – in some units, like Indianapolis, nurses are assigned during the day.

The staff whom the parents and children come into contact with will be doctors, specialist nurses or other professionals who are involved in diagnosing, prescribing, treating, evaluating or teaching (e.g. in diabetic control), who are seen by appointment. They are, no doubt, supportive but are not constantly available.

Parents have been seen as a main source of support, for example in Lexington:

> Also the overwhelming majority of parents found that the presence of other parents and the opportunity to talk with them was helpful – a clearly positive feature of the unit. (Lerner et al 1972)
>
> Mothers also commonly support each other during emotional and stressful periods. (James & Wheeler 1969)

The same is true in Indiana:

> Parents develop formal support groups and some form long-term friendships. (Jennings 1986)

although not in France:

> Parents were to visit only their own child and to refrain from entering other children's rooms; they were not to communicate any medical information, including their PNH (Parenteral Nutrition at Home) experience to their peers. (Brossat & Pinell 1990)

Sometimes parents babysit for each other or help in other ways; in Lexington:

> It is not uncommon to see any or all of the mothers help each other actively, taking

a temperature or baby-sitting while the mother is being interviewed or is out of the hospital for an hour or so, for a walk or a respite. (James & Wheeler 1969)

In Galveston, the rule was tougher:

The parent or other designated care-taker would be responsible for the child at all times while on the unit and this responsibility could not be delegated. (Caldwell 1981).

In Indianapolis, volunteer babysitters were provided so that parents could take a break.

With the careful selection of conditions and the use of strict criteria for admission, there will be little chance of any kind of emergency, so that the absence of medical and nursing staff will not be critical to anyone's survival.

Since there is a limited number of conditions, there can be fairly standard care plans for each as there will be little individual variation.

Flexibility of approach may tend to be less, and if the case deviates from the expected norm, the child will presumably be transferred to conventional care.

The number of children admitted to care-by-parent at any one time will be governed by the number of beds, and admissions will be planned for some time ahead.

In these very structured units, the professionals work in a clearly defined manner, which will reduce stress for them, but parents with 24-hour responsibility in minimally staffed units may find their situation very stressful.

The inclusive approach

Any child with a resident parent may be a candidate for such care and may be admitted to it or transferred at any convenient time.

Care-by-parent will be one of the nursing options available on the wards and not restricted to a particular area or a set number of beds.

The conditions do not need to be specified beforehand but can include anything which is not at a very serious stage; it may also include terminal care for parents who wish to do the caring but feel they cannot cope at home. The child's situation rather than the condition is the determining factor.

When nursing needs are at a level such that the parent can cope with learning, care-by-parent can begin.

When the condition is chronic and requires considerable nursing skills, the process can begin at the earliest appropriate moment: when the parent wishes to take part or the experienced nurse judges that the critical time has arrived. In Jennings' (1988) study, some of the parents who were taking home a child with a tracheostomy felt that they had inadequate opportunity to learn how to change the tube and to develop some confidence before discharge.

With a wide range of conditions, there will be the possibility of deterioration or even emergencies arising, but since they will occur within the ward with regular staff on hand, professional care is immediately available.

If necessary, conventional care can be resumed at little more than a moment's notice without any physical transfer: no little troops of beds and lockers being pushed along corridors.

Flexibility is one of the keynotes of the system. The staff involved in CBP will be part of the regular complement of the ward, although there may be someone with specific responsibility: workload allocation is another question. Similarly, if there is an urgent need for beds, those which have been used for care-by-parent are staffed and part of the resources of the ward.

Parents are available to be taught at any appropriate moment, and staff are there to teach at almost any hour of the day or night. No limit is set beforehand on what can be taught, and the child's needs and the length of stay (which are likely to be related) set the boundaries. There will be sufficient time to teach what is needed, and the transition to responsibility is never abrupt but takes as long as is necessary. Support, reassurance and reinforcement of the teaching are also available from staff, 24 hours a day.

Individualised care plans will be required, as for the other patients, although there will be care elements common to many of them.

This environment will be less stressful for parents because of the constant back-up, but the continual shifting of responsibilities and the range of participation may increase stress for the staff.

Figure 10.3 (p. 142) attempts to compare the two styles of care-by-parent.

The British schemes in Cardiff and Torbay, which have been described, aimed to be inclusive, giving the opportunity of some level of care-by-parent to any child whose condition was not critical and who had a willing parent. They succeeded in doing this for some time, and the results were satisfactory to all the participants (parents, children and professionals), but the effort required to keep them going in the optimum way was not maintained – commitment and continuity were lacking. The flexibility of the system operated against it – any child might or might not be considered for CBP – and the tendency has been to return to familiar ways of working. This seems likely to happen until such time as care-by-parent, like unrestricted visiting and resident parents, has become part of the normal fabric of paediatric nursing from the top down, through its incorporation into policy and nurse education, as well as through gradual changes in ward practice. If change is to be demand-led, perhaps the influence of pressure groups will also be needed.

Until the time comes when parent care is the norm, an inclusive scheme will need someone sufficiently senior to manage it, within wards which have their own ward sisters. At the time of writing, there is no such person in Cardiff and the scheme is at a low ebb. It would be inappropriate for the author to lay down guidelines on how things could be managed, which would in any case depend greatly on the individual hospital and the size and nature of its child patient population. Perhaps, as Chris Bromley has already suggested

	Exclusive	Inclusive
Aims	Better hospital experience for child Improved future for child	
	Learning opportunity for some parents	Optimum learning opportunity for many parents
	Reduced costs	Varies
Hospital	Large	Any with child patients
Area	Separate unit	Ordinary wards
Patients	Specified groups	Any not acutely ill
Criteria	Strictly defined, unproblematic conditions	Individual child and parents, including terminal care
Numbers	Limited by beds	Any bed, no specific limit
Beds	No other use	Used by other patients
Decision	Before admission or transfer, possibly unseen	At any appropriate time, after consideration, seen operating
Admission	Planned	Includes emergencies when stabilised
Staffing	Minimal, possibly non-nursing, day-time only	Professional staff allocated at all times
Professional contact	By appointment	At any time
Teaching	Pre-planned	Anything parent can cope with
Support and reinforcement	Other parents or at staff contact	Mainly staff, other parents may help
Parent care	From admission	Gradual, begins when appropriate
Responsibility	Parents	Shared
Staff stress	Slight	Greater
Parent stress	Greater	Somewhat less

Figure 10.3 Two styles of care-by-parent compared

(Chapter 7), primary nursing would be the model of nursing most sympathetic to care-by-parent.

Exclusive units with restricted aims are an option open to large hospitals whose case load would allow them to plan a viable scheme. They stand a greater chance of success simply because their aims are limited. The range of conditions which could be accommodated would depend on the staff available to them. Experienced qualified nurses could teach what was needed by the parents of children with chronic or long-term conditions, and special groups could be targeted at particular times. If the unit were to be staffed by the new style of support worker, the intake would be limited to those with minimal nursing needs. Resource management might make this an attractive option.

THE IDEAL AND THE REALITY

Experience of care-by-parent in favourable circumstances has demonstrated that it is good for children and satisfying for parents and staff, that the nursing was carried out adequately or better and that no disasters occurred. Nurses were convinced that it reduced the length of stay for many children and made readmission less likely or the need for it better judged. Parents were able to go home with children who would otherwise have spent months, even their whole lives, in hospital, and were able sometimes to cope with death at home. In short, a children's ward which can offer inclusive care-by-parent is ideal. Sadly, ideals may be unattainable, particularly in the face of financial constraints.

Large hospitals may be able to offer care-by-parent to a limited range of children and better learning opportunities to a wider range of parents. In all paediatric units and all wards which nurse children, partnership with the professional rather than paternalism is the keynote of the relationship, and in the words of the standard statement (RCN Paediatric Standards Working Group 1990):

> Parents will be encouraged to be actively involved in the care of their child in hospital

which will (RCN 1991):

> minimise the potentially damaging effects of hospitalisation and promote its therapeutic effects.

REFERENCES

Balint M (1968) *The Doctor, his Patient and the Illness.* London: Pitman.

Ball M, Glasper A & Yerrell P (1988) How well do we perform? Parents' perceptions of paediatric care. *Professional Nurse*, **4**: 115–18.

Bridge J, Bridge S & Luke S (1990) *Blackstone's Guide to the Children Act 1989.* London: Blackstone Press.

Brossat S & Pinell P (1990) Coping with parents. *Sociology of Health & Illness*, **12**: 69–86.

Caldwell BS (1981) A care-by-parent unit. In Azarnoff P & Hardgrove C (eds.), *The Family in Child Health Care*, pp 175–87. New York: Wiley Medical.

Caldwell BS & Lockhart LH (1981) A care-by-parent unit: its planning, implementation and patient satisfaction. *Children's Health Care*, **10**: 4–7.

Clode D, Parker C & Etherington S (eds.) (1987) *Towards the Sensitive Bureaucracy: Consumers, Welfare and the New Pluralism.* Aldershot: Gower.

Coulson D (1988) A proper place for parents. *Nursing Times*, **84**(9): 26–8.

Day A (1987) Can mummy come too? *Nursing Times*, **83**(51): 51–2.

Fisher M (1983) *Speaking of Clients.* Sheffield: University Joint Unit for Social Services Research.

Fradd E (1988) Primary nursing: achieving new roles. *Nursing Times*, **84**(50): 39–41.

Glasper A (1988) Parents in the anaesthetic room: a blessing or a curse? *Professional Nurse*, **3**: 112–15.

Glasper A (1990) A planned approach to nursing children. In Kershaw B & Salvage J (eds.), *Models for Nursing 2*, pp. 89–101. London: Scutari Press.
Glasper A (1992) Personal communication.
Glasper A & Dewar A (1987) Help or hazard? *Nursing Times*, **83**(51): 53–4.
Henderson V (1966) *The Nature of Nursing*. London: Collier-Macmillan.
Hogg C (1989) *The NAWCH Quality Review*. London: NAWCH.
Hooper D (1981) Professional intervention in the parenting process. In Chester R, Diggory P & Sutherland MB (eds.), *Changing Patterns of Child-bearing and Child Rearing*, pp. 167–75. London: Academic Press.
Inman U (1975) *Towards a Theory of Nursing Care*. London: RCN.
James VL & Wheeler WE (1969) The care-by-parent unit. *Pediatrics*, **43**: 488–94.
Jeffery K (1988) *Report on TOPPS*. Unpublished.
Jennings K (1986) Helping them face tomorrow. *Nursing Times*, **82**(4): 33–5.
Jennings P (1988) Nursing and home aspects of the care of a child with tracheostomy. *Journal of Laryngology and Otology*, **Supplement 17**: 25–9.
Kershaw B & Salvage U (1986) *Models For Nursing*. Chichester: John Wiley.
Kitson AL (1989) *Standards of Care – A Framework for Quality*. London: RCN.
Lerner MJ, Haley JV, Hall DS & McVarish D (1972) Hospital care-by-parent: an evaluative look. *Medical Care*, **X**: 430–6.
McFarlane JK (1970) *The Proper Study of the Nurse*. London: RCN.
Monahan GH & Schkade JK (1985) Comparing care by parent and traditional nursing units. *Pediatric Nursing*, **11**: 463–8.
National Institute for Social Work (1988) *Residential Care: a Positive Choice* (The Wagner Report). London: HMSO.
NAWCH (1985) *Charter for Children in Hospital*. London: NAWCH.
NAWCH (1987) *The Emotional Needs of Children Undergoing Surgery*. London: NAWCH.
NAWCH (1988) *Quality Checklist for Caring for Children in Hospital*. London: NAWCH.
Nightingale F (1859) *Notes on Nursing*. Glasgow: Blackie.
RCN (1981) *Towards Standards*. London: RCN.
RCN (1990) *Support Workers – Health Care Assistants*. London: RCN.
RCN (1991) Paediatric Nursing Entities: *Philosophy*. London: RCN.
RCN Paediatric Standards Working Group (1990) *Standards of Care for Paediatric Nursing*. London: RCN.
RCN Society of Paediatric Nursing (1987) *Statement of Values in Paediatric Nursing*. London: RCN.
RCN Working Committee on Standards of Nursing Care (1980) *Setting Standards for Nursing Care*. London: RCN.
Salvage J & Kershaw B (eds.) (1990) *Models for Nursing 2*. London: Scutari Press.
Sidey A (1990) *Family-centred Care at Home*. Paper given at the Conference of the RCN Welsh Paediatric Special Interest Group, Cardiff.
Yura H & Walsh M (1967) *The Nursing Process*. Norwalk CT: Appleton Century Crofts.

FURTHER READING

De'Ath E & Pugh G (eds.) (1988) *Partnership Papers 1–8*. London: National Children's Bureau.

Hadley CM, Dale P & Stacy G (1987) *A Community Social Worker's Handbook*. London: Tavistock Publications.

NAWCH (1987) *The Child Alone: a Report on the Unaccompanied Child in Hospital*. London: NAWCH.

Thornes R (1987) *Where are the Children?* London: Caring for Children in the Health Services, c/o NAWCH.

Thornes R (1988) *Parents Staying Overnight with their Children in Hospital*. London: Caring for Children in the Health Services, c/o NAWCH.

Thornes R (1991) *Just for the Day – Children Admitted to Hospital for Day Treatment*. London: Caring for Children in the Health Services, c/o NAWCH.

Appendix

CONTENTS

- The research methods
- Activity sampling record sheets 1 and 2
- Activity codes
- People codes
- Case study record sheet (part only)
- Nurses' letter and questionnaire
- Letter to all parents and visitors
- Post-discharge questionnaire to CBP parents
- CBP parents' leaflet

THE RESEARCH METHODS

There are problems when young children are the subject of research enquiry. Adults in hospital can be asked to give accounts of what has happened to them and opinions about their treatment. Children, being immature, are less able to comprehend a totally new situation – hospital is a meaningless concept until they get there – or understand the reasons for aspects of their treatment, so they cannot make reliable judgements about their experiences. Their accounts are interesting, especially to the psychologist, but are too subjective to use as data. The very young do not possess the words in which to express themselves, while those older children who do are unlikely to confide in an interviewing stranger.

Staff and relatives can give opinions and accounts of events in which the child has been involved, but these tend to be fragmented and their views are shaped by their own position in and knowledge of the system. The best method for getting information about the life of children in hospital is, therefore, non-participant observation, the 'fly on the wall' technique. The observer records what is going on, remaining unobtrusive, but takes no part in it.

It is sometimes argued that the presence of a watching adult must alter the situation for the child and the staff, but from several hundreds of hours of experience in this role, it appears that this is not the case. The young child accepts the silent observer as just another of the oddities which abound in hospital, one who, thankfully, does nothing to him.

If the observer were approached by a child, the rule was to respond as briefly as possible in a friendly neutral manner, directing him or her to the most appropriate person. To do less would be to alter the situation for the worse. Staff, too, regard the observer as someone unconnected with their own work and go about it in their usual way. The coding was explained to anyone who asked.

Two styles of observation have been used: activity sampling and case study sampling. In both, the observers filled in pre-coded sheets at set intervals (see below for examples of these sheets). The coded observations were supplemented by diaries in which they recorded anything of interest, amplifying the coded material or noting details not covered by it. These methods and the research instruments were based on those used in the earlier Swansea studies of children in hospital.

Activity sampling

Record sheets 1 and 2 (below) represent North Ward and the 8-bedded area of Central Ward schematically, with codes for the state and position of the patients and any action or interaction which was going on. There is space to note the people involved or simply present (these codes are also given below). Observations were made at 20-minute intervals, beginning at 6.15 a.m., 6.20 a.m., 6.25 a.m. or 6.30 a.m., the start time varying so that observations were not made at precisely the same moment each day. The last observations began between 11.15 p.m. and 11.30 p.m. (this was also true of the case studies). At the appropriate time, the observer made a circuit of the two wards, starting at the main door into North Ward, marking down those present and circling the relevant action and interaction codes. People were recorded at the instant they were first seen, not watched for a period, so that what is produced is a series of 'snapshots' rather than a continuous record. This system provided a wealth of data, both qualitative and quantitative, so much so that it could not be computer analysed without losing a vast amount of the detail or spending longer on keying it in than analysing it by hand, which was the conclusion from discussions with several computing advisors in two different institutions. For this reason and the considerable expense of prolonged observations, it seems unlikely that it will be used extensively in the future, but it may provide the basis for more focused techniques of investigation.

Case study sampling

Case study children were observed, with the agreement of their parents, for 5 minutes in each hour. The observer filled in the people codes in a grid, in columns representing 10 seconds (a slot), using a more detailed system of describing interactions, in particular who initiated and who responded. At the end of the 5 minutes, the observer wrote a sentence describing what had happened. Children chosen for case study were either in the Care-by-Parent Scheme when it had been set up or, at the first stage of the observations, would have been suitable for it by reason of their medical condition; not all of them had resident parents. Part of the case study record sheet is included below, showing the categories of action and interaction.

The observers

The observers worked in 4-hour shifts throughout the day, with a half hour overlap in which to get their recording sheets ready and pass on information about admissions and discharges or who were to be the case study children for that day. There were nine observers, five of whom worked at both stages of observation and four at one stage only. They were selected for their experience of children or hospitals: four were teachers, three were nurses (two of whom were also graduates) and the remaining two were a social worker and a physiotherapist. All but one were women hoping to resume their careers after raising their own families. They were trained in the observation techniques by the author, who also acted as an observer.

ACTIVITY SAMPLING RECORD SHEETS 1 AND 2 – *see pages 149 and 150*

ACTIVITY CODES

1. Patient
   - b – baby c – child
   - m – male f – female — Use 1 or 2
2. Emotional state
   - + – happy – – unhappy
   - o – neutral * – angry, aggressive
3. Position
   - D lying Down
   - U sitting Up
   - N standing Near bed
   - A standing Away from bed
   - H being Held, nursed, cuddled
   - M Moving
   - C Carried — Use 1 only
4. Place
   - B Bed or cot
   - P Pram, pushchair, wheelchair

(*continued p. 151*)

Name CP
Time 8.05 a.m.
Date 3.5.84

TV Room (Rachel + M) — **Kitchen**

1. b c m f + o – * Andrea P
D U N A H C M
B P Ch G Op
1 2 3 4 5 6
M SEN (P)
x z c f n p s t
x z c f w (see diary)

4. b c m f + o – * Gary
D U N A H C M
B P Ch G Op
1 2 3 4 5 6 drip monitor
x z c f n p s t
x z c f w

2. b c m f + o – * William P
D U N A H C M
B P Ch G Op Bouncer
1 2 3 4 5 6
M
x z c f n p s t
x z c f w

5. b c m f + o – * Tracey P
D U N A H C M
B P Ch G Op
1 2 3 4 5 6
M blinds down
x z c f n p s t
x z c f w

3. b c m f + o – * Paul
D U N A H C M
B P Ch G Op
1 2 3 4 5 6
x z c f n p s t
x z c f w

6. b c m f + o – *
D U N A H C M
B P Ch G Op
1 2 3 4 5 6
x z c f n p s t
x z c f w

Outside

Corridor 1-6 — 2SN PN A

1. b c m f + o – * Emma
D U N A H C M
B P Ch G Op
1 2 3 4 5 6
x z c f n p s t
x z c f w

5. b c m f + o – * Nicola
D U N A H C M
B P Ch G Op
1 2 3 4 5 6
A (charts)
x z c f n p s t
x z c f w

2. b c m f + o – *
D U N A H C M
B P Ch G Op
1 2 3 4 5 6
x z c f n p s t
x z c f w

6. b c m f + o – * Rachel F
D U N A H C M
B P Ch G Op Bes'n
1 2 3 4 5 6
M
x z c f n p s t
x z c f w

3. b c m f + o – * Jody
D U N A H C M
B P Ch G Op
1 2 3 4 5 6
x z c f n p s t
x z c f w

7. b c m f + o – * Mohammed
D U N A H C M
M's B P Ch G Op
1 2 3 4 5 6
x z c f n p s t
x z c f w

4. b c m f + o – * Sophie
D U N A H C M
B P Ch G Op
1 2 3 4 5 6
x z c f n p s t
x z c f w

8. b c m f + o – *
D U N A H C M
B P Ch G Op
1 2 3 4 5 6
x z c f n p s t
x z c f w

Corridor 7-14 — SN St. SS.

Activity sampling record sheet 1: North Ward

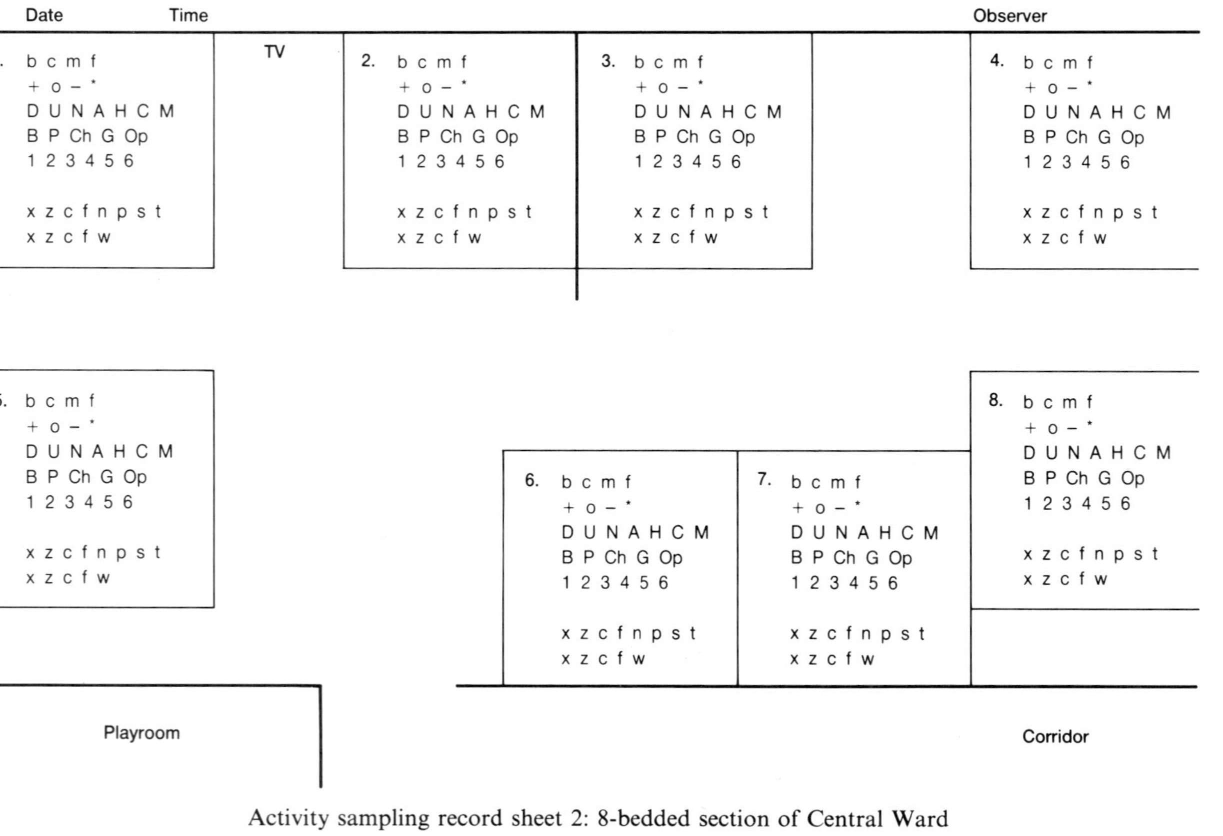

Activity sampling record sheet 2: 8-bedded section of Central Ward

Ch Chair
G Ground, floor
Op Other person
(Other – write in)

5. State
   asleep 1, inactive 2, observant 3,
   active alone 4, alongside 5, with 6.

6. Other present – space for codes.

7. Interaction with child — Several may be used
   x none
   z talk
   c personal care (washing, etc.)
   f food or drink – giving, receiving, consuming
   n nursing care – technical
   p other professional attention, e.g. from physiotherapist or doctor
   s social – generally play
   t touching – patting, holding hand, etc.

8. Interaction between others present
   x none
   z talk
   c personal care
   f food or drink
   w watching

PEOPLE CODES

Case child	√
Other patients – male	m
– female	f
Mother	M
Father	F
Grandmother	GM
Grandfather	GF
Child visitors – male	vm
– female	vf
Other visitors – female	VF
– male	VM

Nurses

Nursing officer Mai Davies	MD
Other nursing officer	NO
Sister	SS
Staff nurse	St

(*continued p. 154*)

CASE STUDY RECORD SHEET (PART ONLY)

Child	1						2		
Time	01–10	11–20	21–30	31–40	41–50	51–60	01–10	11–20	21–30
Place									
0 1 2 3 4 5 6									
emotional state									
Seeks attention									
help, comfort									
specific									
Receives attention									
help, comfort									
praise									
reprimand									
instructions									
gen. comm/n									
food, drink									

wash, bath									
bedpan, etc.									
other person									
bed-make									
medication									
other nursing									
other prof.									
other specific									
Responds attention									
help, comfort									
obeys									
ignores									
specific									
Others present									

Date

Observer

State enrolled nurse	SEN
Student nurse	SN
Pupil nurse	PN
Nursing student	ND
Other learner	N
Auxiliary	A
– add m for male nurse	

Other staff

Doctor – male	Dm
– female	Df
Doctors' round	DR
Receptionist	RNA
Physiotherapist	Ph
Teacher – female	Tf
– male	Tm
Playleader	PL
Other professional	Prof
Medical student	MS
Porter	P
Housekeeping staff	C
Other	O

NURSES' LETTER AND QUESTIONNAIRE

The letter

Department of Child Health
University Hospital of Wales

September 1983

Nursing Children in Hospital

I expect you know by now that research on children in hospital is being carried out in this department. We shall be observing what parents (and other visitors) do for their children and what the children do when they have no visitors.

Obviously having visitors about all the time affects the work on the ward, so we are asking nurses to give us the benefit of their experience and their opinions on the subject. We are interested to know what you think about it, whether you are qualified or a learner, an auxiliary or an RNA. This questionnaire has been prepared and we very much hope that you will fill it in, although it is voluntary, of course.

If you decide to do it, you will find that it does not take very long and I should be glad if you would return it by October 10th. There is an envelope supplied to put it in and you can 'post' it in the boxes in the Sisters' Offices on North and Central Wards. If you prefer, you can hand it to me or to the Child Health Academic Office, or send it through the internal mail.

You can be sure that your answers will be treated in strict confidence – the actual questionnaires will be analysed in Swansea. We should like to have your name on this sheet, which will be detached, in case we want to ask you anything else – but you can leave it off if you prefer. Anyway, I hope you will help.

JEAN CLEARY
Research Officer

Respondent's name. . . . .

The questionnaire

Institute of Health Care Studies
University College Swansea
Nursing Children in Hospital Questionnaire

Please underline or circle the appropriate answer where alternatives are given (if you make a mistake cross it out like this (N̸O̸)); otherwise write your answer in the space provided. Your answer will be entirely confidential and no person's answers will be disclosed to the staff of UHW in any identifiable way.

ID No.
Card No.

1. Are you a qualified nurse? YES NO
   If NO skip to Question 3

2. Are you working for another qualification? YES NO
   If NO skip to Question 6
   If YES skip to Question 8

3. Are you a learner? YES NO
   If YES skip to Question 8

4. Are you an auxiliary nurse? YES NO
   If YES skip to Question 12

5. Are you an RNA? YES NO
   If YES skip to Question 12

Qualified nurses

6. What is your position in the Child Health Department? e.g. Sister, Staff Nurse.

7. What nursing qualifications do you hold? Please list them, with the year in which you gained them.

Now go to Question 12.

Learners

8. What qualifications are you working for? SEN, SRN, RSCN, Degree.

9. What year of training are you in?

10. Do you already hold any other nursing qualifications? YES NO

11. If you do, please list them, with the year in which you gained them.

All

12. What is your age?

    Under 21 31–40
    21–24 41–50
    25–30 51–60

13. How old were you when you left school, Sixth Form or Tertiary College, or College of Further Education (if you went there straight from school)?

14. If you have done other kinds of work apart from nursing, please say what they were.

15. If you have completed any other qualifications or training, please say what they are.

16. If you have nursed outside hospitals or worked for an agency please say
YES NO

What kind of nursing was it and for how long?

17. How long have you worked as a nurse altogether? Give total number of years.

18. How long have you worked in the Child Health Department?

19. Do you have any children of your own? If so, please give their age and sex.

Nursing preferences

20. Which is more important to your satisfaction in your job:
   (i) the people you work with or
   (ii) the patients in the ward?

21. What kind of patients do you most like nursing?

(i) Male, female, no preference.

(ii) Age

Under 1 year	11–15	41–50
1–2 years	16–20	51–60
3–5 years	21–30	61–70
6–10 years	31–40	Over 70
No preference		

Choose as many of these age groups as you wish.

22. What kind of conditions or units do you find most interesting? Again, choose as many as you wish.

1. Paediatrics
2. Obstetrics
3. Special care babies
4. Gynaecology
5. Geriatrics
6. Dermatology
7. Ophthalmology
8. Cardiology
9. Cardiac surgery
10. Neurology
11. Neurosurgery
12. Other medicine
13. Other surgery
14. Out-patients clinic
15. Operating theatres
16. Other (please say what)
17. No preference

Children in hospital

Sometimes questions in this section will refer to children of different ages:

(1) Babies means those less than 1 year old
(2) Small children 1–4 years inclusive
(3) Older children 5–12 years inclusive
(4) Teenagers 13 and over

23. Does your experience suggest that children react differently to being in hospital at different ages? YES NO

24. Excluding those who are extremely ill, or in great pain, would you say that mostly

(1) Babies
- (i) don't really notice where they are
- (ii) are upset by being in hospital
- (iii) just put up with it
- (iv) settle down quickly
- (v) quite enjoy it

(2) Small children
- (i) don't really notice where they are
- (ii) are upset by being in hospital
- (iii) just put up with it
- (iv) settle down quickly
- (v) quite enjoy it

(3) Older children
- (i) don't really notice where they are
- (ii) are upset by being in hospital
- (iii) just put up with it
- (iv) settle down quickly
- (v) quite enjoy it

(4) Teenagers
- (i) don't really notice where they are
- (ii) are upset by being in hospital
- (iii) just put up with it
- (iv) settle down quickly
- (v) quite enjoy it

25. On the whole, do you think that the children on your ward see their parents:

enough, not enough, too much?

26. Considering each group in turn, do you think that *ideally* some relative should:

(1) Babies
- (i) stay in hospital with them
- (ii) visit all day
- (iii) come for a few hours each day
- (iv) come for a few hours most days
- (v) leave it to the staff to look after them?

(2) Small children
(i) stay in hospital with them
(ii) visit all day
(iii) come for a few hours each day
(iv) come for a few hours most days
(v) leave it to the staff to look after them?

(3) Older children
(i) stay in hospital with them
(ii) visit all day
(iii) come for a few hours each day
(iv) come for a few hours most days
(v) leave it to the staff to look after them?

(4) Teenagers
(i) stay in hospital with them
(ii) visit all day
(iii) come for a few hours each day
(iv) come for a few hours most days
(v) leave it to the staff to look after them?

27. Who do you think should stay or visit? Choose as many as you wish: mother, father, grandmother, other relatives (say which):

(1) Babies
(2) Small children
(3) Older children
(4) Teenagers

28. Do you find that you have time to play with bored children or comfort them if they are miserable

(i) mostly
(ii) only at certain times of the day
(iii) rarely
(iv) or feel that it is not really a nurse's job?

29. Do you think that when a child's parents are in the ward they affect the work of the nurse? YES NO
Comment if you would like to.

30. Where
    (1) babies are concerned do you think that their parents
        (i) are a help to the nurse
        (ii) are a hindrance
        (iii) make no difference?

    (2) Small children
        (i) are a help to the nurse
        (ii) are a hindrance
        (iii) make no difference?

    (3) Older children
        (i) are a help to the nurse
        (ii) are a hindrance
        (iii) make no difference?

    (4) Teenagers
        (i) are a help to the nurse
        (ii) are a hindrance
        (iii) make no difference?

31. Do you think that most parents treat their children in the right way while they are in hospital? YES NO

32. Would you say that generally they
    (i) are too strict
    (ii) are too indulgent
    (iii) bring too many presents and too much food
    (iv) play with them sensibly
    (v) don't know what to do
    (vi) encourage too much noise and excitement

    Choose more than one if you wish.

33. It has been suggested that parents might be taught to take over more nursing tasks for their own children, particularly those with chronic conditions. Do you think that this is a good idea? YES NO

34. Here is a list of twenty procedures; would you please tick in the appropriate columns to say whether you think that most, some, or a few parents could be taught to carry them out properly, or whether they should be left to those with professional training.

		Most	Some	Few	Prof. only
1.	General care of the child				
2.	Temperature taking				
3.	Nasogastric tube feeding				
4.	Gastrostomy feeding				
5.	Tracheostomy care				
6.	Care of indwelling catheter				
7.	Post-operative care				
8.	Physiotherapy				
9.	Nasogastric suction				
10.	Stoma care				
11.	Administration of suppositories				
12.	Administration of enemas				
13.	Monitoring infusions				
14.	Taking the apex beat				
15.	MSU				
16.	Gastric intubation				
17.	Wound dressing				
18.	Injections as necessary				
19.	Care of chest drains in situ				
20.	Last offices				

Thank you for taking the time to fill in the questionnaire. If there is any comment you would like to add to the things you have been asked, please use the space below. We should be interested to know whether your own, or your children's, experience of hospital has affected your opinions or even influenced you in choosing a career in nursing.

LETTER TO ALL PARENTS AND VISTORS

Research on children in hospital

To parents and other visitors,

Visiting children in hospital has changed considerably over the past twenty-five years; visitors now can be with their children in the University Hospital for as long as they choose and are doing more and more to look after their children.

In this Child Health Department, the medical and nursing staff are cooperating with social scientists to find out how these changes have altered life on the ward. The information will help decide whether any other changes are needed.

For the next few weeks, observers on North and Central Wards will record how children, their visitors and the staff spend their time. They are not here to assess what is done in any way. There is no need to take notice of them as they go round – just carry on as though they weren't there. You may not even notice that they *are* there.

Some of the time the observers will be looking at the whole ward, at others they will study a particular child (not one who is seriously ill) for five minutes at a stretch.

If you would like to find out more about the research, Mrs Cleary will be happy to talk to you about it. If for any reason you do not wish to join in this important study, we will, of course, respect your decision.

Professor OP Gray (Head of Department)
Miss Mai Davies (Nursing Officer)
Mrs Jean Cleary (Research Officer)

POST-DISCHARGE QUESTIONNAIRE TO CBP PARENTS

University College of Swansea: Institute of Health Care Studies.

Post-hospital Questionnaire

1. Name
4. Hospital No.
2. Date of birth
5. Age at admission
3. Address
6. House, flat, part, shared accommodation
7. Household composition
8. Length of stay
9. Continuous, leave, readmission
10. Care-by-parent – how long?

Previous experience

11. Has s/he been in hospital before?
12. Admission planned/emergency
route – parent, GP-h, GP-s, OP, ward
13. Were you expecting admission?

Hospital experience

14. How ill was s/he on admission?

15. What were the symptoms?

16. Did you intend to stay anyway?

17. Who stayed? M, F, both, alternating, mainly M
    Specify any other

18. Other children

19. How have you managed?

20. Did being in hospital cause extra expense?

Fares/petrol	Meals in hospital
New clothing	Care for other children
Presents	Time off work Mother
	Father
Other	

21. Could you estimate the total cost?

22. Are you working?
    Looking for work?

23. Is there a male breadwinner in the family?
    What is his job?
    Is he employed at the moment?
    If not, how long?

Baby

24. Do you think that was old enough to notice anything different about being in hospital?

25. Is s/he normally: happy/miserable/wants attention?
    sleeps well/badly?
    feeds well/badly?

26. How did s/he behave in hospital?

27. At home again – back to normal straightaway?
problems
or improvements? feeding
sleeping
clinging
crying more
more contented
livelier
not really recovered yet

Child

28. Do you think that was old enough to
notice the difference
at first too ill to care
upset by it
contented while M or F, other there
settled down quickly

29. Is normally
happy/miserable
quiet, active
adventurous/stays close

30. Does s/he eat
well/badly
sleep well/badly

31. How did s/he behave in hospital?

32. After going home, back to normal?
straightaway, soon, not yet?
problems or
improvements? feeding
sleeping
clinging
more independent
bad tempered
better-tempered
aggressive

33. Was it possible to explain anything?

34. Have you talked about it since going home?

Care-by-parent nursing

35. Which of these did you do in hospital or do at home?

	HOSPITAL				HOME
	Nurses	Attempt	Did	Charted	B/A
i. take temperature					
ii. respiration					
iii. pulse					
iv. fluid intake					
v. urine collection					
vi. medication oral					
vii. nasogastric feed					
viii. medication					
ix. pass tube					
x. drip check					
change bag					
xi. oxygen tent					
mask					
xii. mist tent					
xiii. nebuliser					
xiv. chest suction					
xv. stoma care					
xvi. physiotherapy					
xvii. other					

36. Did you accompany to X-ray or operating theatre?

37. Did s/he have blood tests?
biopsy?
injections?
other?

Parents' opinions of care-by-parent

38. Good idea, would do again?
too much of a tie?
too much responsibility?

39. How did you arrange your own breaks?

40. What did you think of the facilities for parents' meals, sleeping etc?

41. How soon was care-by-parent mentioned to you?

42. Who by?

43. How long did it take you to make up your mind?

Information and procedures

44. Do you think that the system was explained well beforehand?

45. Did you find the booklet adequate?

46. Were there problems finding the right nurse
getting information

47. Did you ever find that a nurse had done something, eg. temperature, that you were going to do, without checking with you first?

48. Was TPR explained well, too much expected too quickly?

49. Were the nurses who explained sympathetic, patient?

50. How many were involved in teaching you?

51. Did you find the other mothers friendly?

52. Did they help with information about things on the ward?
in the hospital?

53. Did they show you how to do things eg. temperature, or help you with them?

54. Do you feel that your confidence in dealing with illness has increased?

55. Would you take temperatures, etc. at home?

56. Do you think that you could learn other things, eg. nasogastric tube, injections?

CBP PARENTS' LEAFLET

Introduction to the Care-by-Parent Scheme

The staff of the University Hospital of Wales believe that it is most important to avoid separation of children and their parents more than can be avoided, especially when they are ill and their mothers and fathers can play an important part in looking after their child while in hospital. A Care-by-Parent Scheme has been running since May 1984 and has been found extremely worthwhile. If you wish to care for your child, you will be shown what to do by the nurses who look after your child, while he/she is here. What you learn will help you to keep your child as healthy as possible and to know what to do if he/she is similarly ill at home. Children are less likely to be upset by being in hospital when cared for by parents or relatives.

Medical care

One of the consultant paediatricians has general overall responsibility for your child's treatment. A senior doctor will be responsible for the day-to-day medical care of your child.

Nursing care

There will always be (at least) one Care-by-Parent nurse whose job it is to look after children who are in the Care-by-Parent Scheme. They help parents and answer their questions. They wear a badge similar to that outside the cubicle.

What parents can do

The parents of all children in the unit do the usual things for their children, as far as possible, like feeding, bathing and changing, looking after them, and playing with them as they would at home.

Parents in the Scheme take part in the nursing care of the child in addition. The Care-by-Parent nurse shows parents what to do, e.g. to take temperature and record it on the chart or give medicine, and helps until they feel confident about doing it themselves.

Do not worry about asking to be shown something again; the nurse will not expect you to be an expert straight away. Each child is assessed individually and the mother or father is taught what is necessary, such as collecting urine specimens or giving nasogastric (tube) feeds. Parents go with their children to other hospital departments for tests or treatments and generally stay with them while the tests are carried out. If you prefer not to accompany your child, don't hesitate to let the nurse know beforehand. Don't be afraid to admit you cannot manage some aspect of your child's condition.

Meals for patients

Babies can usually carry on with the milk they have at home, and there is a wide selection of milk feeds and baby food available on the ward. Special diets are supplied via the dietetic department.

Children's meals can generally be selected from the daily menu, by the parents, and are served at the following times:

Breakfast	7.30 a.m.
Lunch	12.00 midday
Supper	5.30–6.00 p.m.

Drinks for children are freely available within the ward, e.g. milk, tea, coffee, fruit drinks, etc.

The hospital aims to provide a balanced diet, so we hope you will not give too many extras, e.g. sweets or crisps.

Important: Do not give sweets, etc. to other children in the unit; they may be on special diets or having to go without for a particular reason – like before an anaesthetic.

Facilities for parents

Resident parents have to pay for their own meals, but they are allowed to use the staff restaurant. They (and other visitors) can also use the Lakeside Centre, which is open on weekdays:

Breakfast	7.30 a.m. – 11.00 a.m.
Lunch	12.00 midday – 2.00 p.m.
Supper	5.30 p.m. – 7.30 p.m.

Drinks and snacks can also be obtained from WRVS counters in:

the hospital concourse;
the paediatric out-patients;
the main out-patients.

There is a parents' lounge on North Ward with a TV set. Adjoining it there is a kitchen where you can make tea or coffee and a parents' bathroom and toilet.

Daily activities

Children are woken about 7.00 a.m. and are expected to be washed or bathed and dressed before or after breakfast. They can wear either their own clothes or ones provided by the hospital.

Parents should be up by 9.00 a.m.

Children of school age, who are well enough, attend the hospital school. There are two full-time teachers. For the younger children there is a playleader who helps with toys and games that can be played within the cubicles if necessary. There are baby-walkers and baby-bouncers, too.

It is a good idea to take babies and children out for walks if possible, and prams are available in the unit. Let the nurse know where you are going before you take patients out of the ward – tell her, too, if you are going for a meal or a break and want the staff to take over while you are away.

Sick children need extra rest and being in hospital is a strain on parents, too, so we advise early bedtimes, even though this may not be your habit at home.

What to bring for your child

Children can wear their own day and night clothes; hospital clothes are available, if needed. The hospital launders hospital clothes; your own can either be washed at home or in the unit's washing machine – but you must provide your own washing powder.

Bring dressing gown, shoes and slippers and your child's toilet things – soap, flannel, toothbrush and paste, brush and comb. The hospital will provide towels.

Bring favourite toys, books or games, but make sure they are clearly marked. There is a bedside locker for keeping your child's things in.

What to bring for yourself

Bring comfortable day and night clothes and shoes. Remember that the wards are usually very warm.

Stiletto heels damage flooring, so we hope you and your visitors will avoid wearing these.

Bring toilet things and towels for yourself, and books, knitting, etc. to help you pass the time. There will be a small cupboard for you to keep your clothes, etc. in whenever possible.

The hospital cannot accept responsibility for the loss of money, valuables or clothing, etc., so we advise you to keep the minimum you need in your room.

Parents' accommodation

Only one parent can be accommodated in the cubicle with the child. A folding bed is provided. There is no room for brothers and sisters to stay (except for a breast-fed baby). In exceptional circumstances, e.g. a critically ill child, the nursing staff can arrange for both parents to be accommodated.

There is a sitting room with an adjoining kitchen, bathroom and toilet for parents' use. It is not intended for other visitors. Smoking is **not permitted** in this area.

Housekeeping

A ward housekeeper will clean your child's room once a day, but parents are expected to keep it tidy.

Smoking

We realise that parents who smoke do so particularly when they are anxious. However, smoking is a health hazard, not only to the smoker but also to those around, particularly sick children or babies; there is also the danger of accidental fire. Smoking cannot be permitted anywhere in the ward. It is permitted *only* in the area provided in the unit entrance hallway, in the concourse, or the general out-patients waiting area.

Visiting

Parents not involved in the Care-by-Parent Scheme can visit at any time. Other children can come with their parents, but responsibility for their safety and behaviour rests with the parents. Unruly children will have to be taken home. Children are expected to behave in a suitable manner for a hospital where there are very sick children.

Other visitors are welcome, but do not encourage too many to come at once; a sick child can find it very tiring and may prefer to be quiet. Remember the other patients, too. Visitors other than parents should leave the ward by 8 p.m. Special visiting arrangements can always be made with the nursing staff.

Telephones

Relatives who want news of a child's progress can telephone the hospital at:

Cardiff 755944; ask for
North Ward, Paediatric Unit.

There are two public telephones in the unit entrance hallway (outgoing calls only) as well as several in the concourse.

Other facilities

In the concourse there are several shops which can be used by visitors. There is a newsagent's which sells a variety of other goods (not tobacco), a flower and fruit shop and a hairdresser's which sells toiletries. There is a post office and a branch of NatWest Bank.

Religion

The hospital chapel is situated on the 5th floor of B Block and is always open to patients and visitors. The services of hospital chaplains are available at all times. Ministers of all denominations can be contacted via the nursing staff. Your own minister of religion can visit you and your child at any time.

Social work department

Contact can be made with this department through the nursing staff whenever necessary.

Ideas and complaints

The Care-by-Parent Scheme is new in Britain and we welcome ideas to help it work. We are also interested in suggestions which would make the child's or parents' stay more pleasant.

We welcome comments upon your child's care or your stay straight away or on discharge, so they can be considered as soon as possible. Please tell the Ward Sister or the Unit Nursing Officer of any problems before taking your child home.

Index

accidents 8
accommodation, parental 9, 13, 20, 74, 134
activity 22–7
  in corridor 24–5
  patterns 23
  sampling 21, 147
admissions 3, 8, 13, 121–2
  elective 98, 130
  emergency 98, 131
  procedures 98
adolescents 134
adult wards 7, 39
advocacy 128
ages, rate of admission 4
alone on ward 10, 27, 52
ambivalence, to parents 111
anaesthesia 1, 27, 34
antisepsis 1
anxiety 13, 14, 69
apnoea 58–9, 104
asthma 4, 19, 35, 79
attachment 2, 58
attitude to care-by-parent 72–3, 80

babysitters, volunteer 121, 140
barrier nursing 12, 52, 71
basic care 20
bed utilisation 114
behaviour problems 9, 14, 70, 120
boredom
  children 10
  parents 13, 39, 71
Bowlby, John 2, 54, 58
breaks, parental 73–4
Bromley, Chris 93, 95

cancer 4; *see also* oncology, paediatric
Caps 44, 95
Cardiff Scheme 15, 19–35, 38–46, 48–66, 96
care-by-parent 15, 37
  admissions to 119
  benefits 122–3
  costs to parents 75–6
  criticisms 89–91
  criteria 119–21
  developments 97, 105–6
  economics of 123
  financial benefits 69
  leaflet 170–4
  planning 137–8
  setting up 37–46
  staff experience 15–16
  US experience 37, 114–25
care-by-parent nurse 43, 44, 77–8
care, individualised 130–2
care model, family-centred 110, 130
care, nature of 54–8
care of other children 27–9, 75

care plan 99–102, 141
case assignment 12, 57
case study sampling 147
cerebral palsy 19
chest infection 42, 51
child's experience 12
childcare 2
Children Act 1989 127, 128
children's hospitals 2
chronic conditions 4
cognitive development 12
comfort 54
commitment 138
communication 76, 132
community health services 133
community paediatric nursing 14
competence, parental 14, 78, 115
confidence 78, 115
confusion 78
congenital heart disease 19, 46, 103
contacts 21, 54
  patterns 30–2, 54
continuity of care 30, 138
Court Report 3, 7
crying 29, 52–4
curriculum 108–9
  hidden 109, 111
  planned 109–11
  unplanned 111
cystic fibrosis 4, 35, 42, 71, 79, 120

Davies, Carole 93
Davies, Mai 38, 87, 89, 93
day-care 3
diabetes 3, 19, 38, 42, 79, 120, 121
diarrhoea 60, 120
disability 127
discharges 6
distraction 46
disturbance, post-hospital 10, 14
doctors' attitude to care-by-parent 91
domiciliary paediatric nursing 3, 133, 136

eating 34; *see also* feeding; meals
Eden, Carol 88, 93
education 121
  disrupted 10
  see also hospital school
emotional need 1
environment, physical 12, 51
exclusive approach 138–40; *cf.* inclusive approach

failure to thrive 42, 46
fathers 13, 75
febrile convulsions 42, 102–3
feeding 34, 54, 55
  problems 120
  see also nasogastric feeding
Ferguson, Marion 38, 39, 40
flexibility 141
friendships 26, 33

gate-keepers 128, 139
gastro-enteritis 19, 42, 46, 50
Gray, Peter 39, 42, 46
Green, Morris 37, 96, 117, 123–5
guidelines, Care-by-Parent 98
guilt 13

haemophilia 38
Hall, David 40
hernia 19
'hidden' children 6
hidden curriculum 109, 111
hospital school 20
hospitalisation
  effects of 1, 8, 38
  experience 11–13
  non-damaging 9
  long-stay 11–12
  rates 4
hydrocephalus 5, 19, 51, 62–5

immunisation 2
inclusive approach 140–2; *cf.* exclusive approach
informal support 117
information 76
involvement, parental 14–15, 130

James Whitcomb Riley Hospital 116, 117
Jeffery, Karen 135, 136
job satisfaction 39, 91

kidney disease 42
Körner system 4

language, expressive 34, 117
Lee, Ming Shu 80
life in the ward 19–35, 48–68
loneliness 27, 35
long-stay patients 10, 11–12

maturity 34
meals 74; *see also* feeding
medication 121
  responsibility for 135
metabolic disorders 5, 46
mobility 34
monitoring 132
multiple handling 2, 39

nasogastric feeding 20, 38, 60, 88, 104
nasopharyngeal suction 60, 61, 78, 104
NAWCH 9
NAWCH Charter 128
North American units 96
nurses' attitudes 9, 83–93
Nurses' Questionnaire 83–6, 155–63
nurses' role 109
nursing developments 128–9
nursing procedures 86
nursing skill and parents 38

oncology, paediatric 19
observations 20, 35, 48–9
observers 41, 148

parent/staff relationships 78
parents
  attitudes 80
  breaks 73
  experience 13, 68–81
  facilities 39, 74
  involvement 14, 79
  meals 73–4
  needs 20, 121
  and nursing procedures 86
  participation 115
  resident 3, 13
  role 58–9
  of teenagers 85
  visiting 3
  on the ward 85–6
  see also accommodation; care-by-parent; fathers
partnership 108
  cycle 115
patient care 42
patient, long-stay 10, 11–12
patient/staff relationships 34, 109
personal care 34, 54, 57
Perthes' disease 12
philosophy of care 15, 41, 108–13
physiotherapy 38
  by parent 35
planned curriculum 109–10
planning 137–8
Platt Committee 1, 3
Platt Report 7, 19, 127
  recommendations 3
  outcome 39
play 32–4, 54; *see also* therapeutic play
playleaders 10, 20, 32, 34
Post-Discharge Questionnaire 72, 164–69
PREPP 133
pressure area care 38
primary nursing 12, 90, 105–6
Project 2000 112–13, 133
psoriasis 35
psychological needs 3, 20, 45, 117
psychosocial factors 9
public health 1

Quality Checklist 132–3

readmissions 3–6
research 9
  methods 146
resources
  management 142
  utilisation 114
responsibility 73, 121
  for medication 135
  parental 136
Robertson, James 2, 45

Sainsbury, Clive 93, 135
safety 130
Saunders, Jaqueline 92
school attendance 20, 26–7, 121; *see also* hospital school
selection for Care-by-Parent 41–3
separation 2, 12
'sightings' 21
sleep patterns 22–3
sleeping 51
smoking 20, 26, 106
social interaction 32, 34, 54–8
  between parents 35
social needs 1, 3
Southampton Scheme 136
special needs of adolescents 134
spina bifida 4, 38
Stacey, Margaret 9, 38, 39, 40

staff experience of Care-by-Parent 15
standards 112, 129–34
stimulation 51, 57
stress 140–1
students 112–13, 114
surgery 8
Swansea studies 9–11

talk as social need 54
teaching 44–5, 78, 97, 136, 141
telephone use 26
television 22, 29–32, 35
terminal care 103, 140
therapeutic play 117, 121
Thornes, Rosemary 6, 96
toileting 20, 34, 45
TOPPS 135
Torbay Scheme 93, 135, 141
Toronto Scheme 39
total care 90
tracheostomy 38, 42, 78, 119

unplanned curriculum 111
urinary infection 42
US experience 37, 114–23

value clarification 112
Vancouver Scheme 39, 123
visiting
  parental 130
  patterns 30
  restricted 2, 39
  unrestricted 3, 8, 9, 10, 13
vulnerability 10

ward attenders 6
ward environment 141; *see also* environment, physical
ward management 102
ward routine 20, 35
washing 20, 45; *see also* toileting
work ethic 111
Welfare of Children in Hospital (Platt Report) 1, 3, 95–6
Welfare of Children and Young People in Hospital 1991 134
worry 71